Early praise from the medical communit

D0360776

"Completely engaging and full of useful ideas [   ] struggled with a weight problem. I could not put it down. *Doctor's Orders* shows how a revolution of weight loss treatments and technology has taken place and how anyone can take advantage of it with Dr. Sasse's clear and straightforward advice. This is the best weight loss book in print today."

—*Martin Bain, MD, Fellow of the American College of Surgeons*

"An extremely powerful and effective resource containing the most powerful tools for effective long-term weight loss. Dr. Sasse goes far beyond the scientific details and provides an all-encompassing, simple-to-follow, guide for weight-loss success. Written by one of the foremost experts in the medical weight loss field, *Doctor's Orders* is an absolutely essential guide for anyone wishing to lose weight."

Stephen B. Mayville, Ph.D., B.C.B.A.
Licensed Clinical Psycholgist
Board Certified Behavior Analyst

"Delightful and entertaining, Dr. Sasse has managed to inform, inspire, and illuminate with a well-researched and well-written book about the changing world of weight loss treatment. Each of us needs to read this book to maintain our waistlines and improve our health. This is a book that I will enthusiastically recommend to all my patients, colleagues and friends!"

—*Gayl Fording, RN*

"*Doctor's Orders* is the prescription for making those lifestyle changes to lose weight and keep it off. Every tip is a nugget of information proven to help you reach your goals. Every page gives you a small, manageable step to get you on track for success. Forget the complicated diet books. Follow *Doctor's Orders* and you'll see results on the scale and feel better than you have for a long time."

—*Vicki Bovee, MS, RD, professional Dietitian and Co-author,*
Ditch Your Diet in 90 Days

"Highly readable, fun, and thought-provoking, *Doctor's Orders* gives us all what we have truly needed: one simple expert resource with proven successful techniques for weight loss. This is a resource that should be on every bookshelf at home and at every doctor's office."

—*Dr. Wes Hall, MD*

"Finally, a practical weight-loss guide that brings the proven science to the real world of daily living and daily decisions. I can say with the upmost confidence that if you follow even some of Dr. Sasse's proven Tips, you will lose weight and become healthier."

—*Kevin Lasko, MD physician and weight loss patient*

"Dr. Sasse's common sense and informative approach makes this the best weight loss book I have ever read! This is the only book on weight loss you will ever need to read."

Phillip E. Dahan, M.D., C. M., F.A.C.S.
Plastic & Reconstructive Surgeon
Certified by the Royal College of Physicians and Surgeons of Canada
McGill University, Montreal, Canada

"WOW!! TRULY a wealth of knowledge and experience was put in to this book. I will use it to hand out to my Life Coaching clients who are working to lose weight and improve their health. Thank you for putting this together - it certainly makes my job easier to hand this book out to my weight loss clients considering a new path in their health and happiness with weight loss. It is a must read for anyone ready to jump start their weight loss. Not only is his book an easy-to-follow guide and knowledge manual, but it also inspires the reader to see how they CAN DO IT and how they WILL SUCCEED! The world has changed, and the tools are there for a person to succeed with weight loss, at long last. I commend Dr. Sasse for compiling his wealth of knowledge and experience into this book for giving so many people hope."

—*Richard Cunningham, Professional Life Coach*

Doctor's Orders:
101 Medically-Proven Tips For Losing Weight

A SASSE GUIDE™

Kent Sasse, MD, MPH, FACS

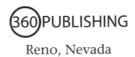
360 PUBLISHING
Reno, Nevada

360° Publishing, LLC.
3495 Lakeside Drive
Suite 205
Reno, NV 89509
www.sasseguide.com

Book Cover and Page Layout: Anita Jones, Another Jones Graphics

ISBN: 978-1-934727-22-5

Visit Dr. Sasse's website at www.sasseguide.com

Publisher's Cataloging-In-Publication Data
(Prepared by The Donohue Group, Inc.)

Sasse, Kent.
    Doctor's orders : 101 medically-proven tips for losing weight / Kent Sasse.

    p. : ill. ; cm. -- (Sasse guide)

    Includes bibliographical references and index.
    ISBN: 978-1-934727-22-5

1. Weight loss--Popular works. 2. Reducing diets--Popular works. 3. Reducing exercises--Popular works. I. Title.

RM222.2 .S27 2009
613.2/5

This book is dedicated to my patients who are my real teachers and sources of inspiration.

Foreword ix

Introduction..xi

Medically-Proven Tips for a New You................................1

  A Day in the Life 3
  The Goal: Setting Goals 21
  Fueling and Refueling: Food 49
  The Working Life..69
  The Working-Out Life 75
  Food for Thought...91
  Bonus Tips 99
  Conclusion..105

Appendices

  A – Recipes 109
  B – Liquid Diet Replacement Plan 125
  C – Body Mass Index (BMI) 127
  D – Work Out Plans 128
  E – Rebound Weight Gain Blamed for Diets Failing...133
  F – References...135

Resources...141
About the Author..155
Index of Tips by Chapter 157
Other books..162

Nearly 60 years ago a new field of medicine appeared, one that focused on the human condition of excessive weight and obesity. A small group of Osteopathic physicians in 1950 formed the first medical society dedicated to the study and treatment of excessive weight and obesity and named this national medical society the 'Glandular Society' in part due to their belief that obesity and in particular morbid obesity had a glandular or hormonal component to its cause or etiology.

I would have never thought when I entered the field of medicine known as bariatric medicine in the 1980s, or even nearly two decades later in 2000 while serving on the board of directors to what then became the American Society of Bariatric Physicians that we would have learned so much about the cause and treatment of obesity. Until now these medical advancements have done little to stem the explosive growth of our nation's obesity epidemic. We have needed more effective, easily applied and scientifically-based Tips and guidelines that can be integrated in our day-to-day living to produce weight loss without great stress or anxiety.

I believe that Dr. Sasse, one our foremost experts in the field of obesity medicine and surgery, has brought us these essential and easily followed guidelines that can not only help us lose weight but bring about long-term weight loss. Until now, I've found no single book or resource which has pulled together in a concise and applicable way all of the proven treatment modalities which have stood the test of time along with the latest that science has to offer in a simple, straightforward and practical guide. That is exactly what Dr. Sasse has done here with *Doctor's Orders: 101 Medically Proven Tips for Losing Weight.*

This book offers an impressive collection of medically-proven weight loss tips and tools. They are simple to follow, easy, and remarkable in the success they bring to your weight loss efforts. Never before has such a weight-loss guide been so grounded in the scientific research of what really works in our day to day lives. For anyone seeking to lose weight, from a few pounds to a few hundred pounds, this book is essential reading

Dr. Sasse breaks new ground with this exciting and novel new book compiling medically-proven weight loss tips into one succinct and easy to follow, easy to read and entertaining guideline. His candor, sense of humor, clarity and practicality have the power to help millions of people lose weight and maintain that weight loss.

If you read only one book about how to lose weight, this is it.

Kevin Huffman, DO
Medical Director
American Bariatric Centers
www.americanbariatricconsultants.com

Why I Wrote This Book for You

I wrote this book to help you lose weight and improve your life, pure and simple. As a physician and surgeon specializing in the care of overweight patients, I wrote this book to introduce people to the best available medically-proven weight-loss treatments, tools and techniques.

To serve the growing number of people with health problems related to being severely overweight, I founded and helped establish a surgical weight-loss center that has grown and developed an outstanding national reputation. Along the way, I discovered a great many medically proven tips and techniques that can help *everyone* who needs to lose weight, not just those undergoing surgery.

After researching how best to serve my overweight patients who were embarking upon a surgical weight-loss journey, our center, Western Bariatric Institute, implemented a number of highly successful programs to ensure that each patient would have the greatest odds of long-term success. This started immediately with an intensive medically guided pre-surgery weight-loss program. Most patients quickly lost 20 to 30 pounds on the four-week intensive program, which became the basis of the **How to Lose 40 Pounds in 90 Days Safely** audio CD and induction medical weight-loss program.

Our medically supervised weight-loss program emphasizes intensive education to provide each patient the tools necessary to change behaviors and create healthy long-term habits. These habits and behavior tools are focused on easy-to-incorporate tips for everyday life. The program includes specific medical advice on setting goals, choosing fun and healthy activities to get active and lose weight and selecting the right foods. It covers medically proven tips for weight loss at work, utilizing ongoing support groups, choosing the right exercise regimen and help with planning, staying motivated, improving mindfulness and even eating healthier at restaurants.

Our extensive experience with medically-supervised weight loss led to the identification of the key tips and techniques that work the best for weight-loss success. This book contains more than 101 valuable ideas, tips and bits of knowledge that can change your life. Integrating these tips into your life will help you achieve your goals of losing weight and becoming a healthier new you. I wish you great success in your weight-loss journey.

Medically Proven Tips for a New You

It's choice – not chance- that determines your destiny.

—Jean Nidetch

A Day in the Life

Every day of your weight-loss journey you make hundreds of small choices that determine whether you will succeed in losing weight or continue to slowly gain. Looking at the way you make those tiny, day-in-the-life decisions and making changes so each decision favors improved health and weight loss isn't difficult once you get started.

The key is to remember that small changes become BIG changes when you multiply their effect over 365 days. Small, almost insignificant, alterations in your activities and daily routines may increase the calories you burn by only 10, 20 or 50 calories a day. But make three or four of those "insignificant" changes, and then multiply their effect over 365 days, and you have lost a lot of pounds! This is what I call the multiplier effect.

Unfortunately, the multiplier effect works both ways. If you work in an office with a candy bowl and you dip in a few times a day, eating three or four pieces throughout the work day, that's no big deal, right? Not quite: Those treats add at least an extra 100 calories per day to your daily total intake. That's not too bad. But bring in the multiplier effect and now you have five days a week and 52 weeks a year. That's an extra 24,000 calories each and every year, around seven pounds every year. No wonder most Americans gain five to 10 pounds every year after age 40!

> ### The Multiplier Effect
> You cut out one daily bite of a cookie or candy bar: 50 calories
> Multiply by 365 days a year: 18,250 calories
> This means losing FIVE pounds every year.

1. Eat breakfast every morning

Eating breakfast turns on the metabolism and helps us burn more calories throughout the day.

It sounds simple, but it may not be. For some reason, eating breakfast has been one of the hardest habits for me (and for many of my patients) to establish. I used to get up, shower, dress and head to work with no nutritional input for a good three or four hours. I have numerous colleagues who start their days with nothing more than a cup of coffee. A lot of people just don't feel hungry in the morning. Unfortunately, skipping

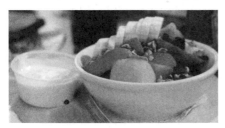

breakfast usually leads to consuming more calories later in the day and into the evening, a pattern that leads to increased storage of fat and, as a result, weight gain.

Get in the habit of eating breakfast. Any new habit only takes a couple weeks to become automatic and maybe even pleasant: a quiet time before the day begins.

The trick is to get in the healthy breakfast habit. Quick, easy, unhealthy breakfast options abound, from doughnuts in the boardroom to fast-food sandwiches at the drive-through, and many of these options are full of fat and carbohydrates.

Breakfast is the perfect time of day for a healthy protein bar. The best contain somewhere in the neighborhood of 150 to 230 calories and 12 to 15 grams of protein with very few carbo-hydrates, probably less than 10. And a protein bar is as simple as a doughnut: This kind of breakfast needs no preparation, no cooking, no cleaning. It fills you up and fuels you up, satis-fies your appetite and doesn't trigger the hormonal surges of blood glucose insulin and leptin (another important regulatory metabolic hormone) that lead to weight gain and more hunger (commonly known as a "sugar rush," which ultimately leads to a crash anyway.) If you have time, and you like to cook, try to mimic this nutritional content, but avoid the tall glass of juice with the muffin.

While this particular breakfast—juice and muffin or pastry—might seem healthy to some, in light of what we've learned about low-carbohydrate diets, this particular breakfast is nothing but a lot of carbohydrates plus a bit of fat. The refined flour in a muffin provides enough simple carbohydrate for days and the juice serves only to further trigger surges of blood glucose, insulin and leptin. It's not only unhealthy, it will be quickly absorbed and leave you hungry again within a very short amount of time, and therefore in danger of making other bad food choices. Breakfast is an important meal. Don't squander your calories and start the day off this way!

2. Set short-term goals

How many pounds do you want to lose in the next month? Write it down. Be realistic as well as optimistic. Try picking other short-term goals, too, like working out every weekday, weighing yourself every morning or avoiding desserts for the entire week. Attainable short-term goals can buoy you up for longer term goals. No one can accomplish a vast, long-term objective all at once. It takes time and baby steps, planned out in detail. Write those steps down and stick to them.

3. Find rewards other than food

Once you start attaining those goals, find ways to reward yourself that don't involve a food treat. Massages, good books, movies, clothes, even just some time to relax, are all treats on their own. Use your imagination. Think of people you like to visit with or long-distance friends you haven't talked to on the phone for a while. Think of that hybrid rose you've been wanting to buy and treat yourself to it, as well as the time to enjoy planting it. Give yourself small rewards and celebrate small successes along the way.

4. Park farther away

Park at least an extra two rows away from the entrance to your work. Or the entrance to your gym or grocery store or any other place you routinely visit. It's a win-lose proposition: You win by saving time (because you're not randomly, repeatedly circling the parking lot, trying to get closer) and you lose—pounds.

The key here is sustainability. Two extra rows might not seem like much, and that's a good thing: How hard is it simply to walk that small distance? It's an easy habit to get into. Do the math: Burning an additional 50 calories a day by parking and walking can add up to 18,250 calories over the course of a year. That translates into more than five pounds lost each year, just from one little change.

There's even a green component to this plan: Think about the gas you won't use circling the parking lot and the pollutants your car won't expend.

You might even enjoy it. There may be landscaping around the office you've never appreciated or neighbors you meet on the way into the neighborhood grocery who you might otherwise not meet. In my case, there's a gorgeous sycamore outside the entrance to one of the hospitals where I practice. It's a bit out of my way, but I make a point to pass it as often as I can, which adds 100 steps to my routine. both coming and going, and enriches my day.

5. Take the stairs

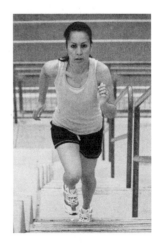

Going up only one level? Take the stairs. Think of the benefits—you don't have to wait for the elevator or spend the ride in cramped quarters with strangers who don't share your tastes in body odor or cologne. One flight of stairs can burn approximately 16 calories and it will probably get you there faster than the elevator can. Make it a habit.

Stairs are physically challenging. Startling your body into suddenly expending energy to climb up a flight of stairs causes almost anyone to breathe hard. And sometimes physical limitations prevent you from climbing stairs. If so, there are more than 100 other tips in this book—and maybe a chance those stairs can become attainable.

6. Fight back when the day gets crazy

Some days just don't fall into line, no matter how well you plan. The day turns crazy. The kids need something. A crisis happens at work. Unexpected events cancel your well-planned lunch and dinner regimen.

What can you do to avoid the binge that can happen if you go too long without feeding the beast?

Keep some low-carb snacks available. Some of the protein bars don't hold up well in the car in the summer heat, but others do. Experiment and try stashing a box of the kind that are not covered in chocolate somewhere in your car.

Then think of some other snacks that work for you: beef jerky, cheese sticks and other low-carb snacks, and keep them available for when the day falls apart, you're out running errands and there is no way to have an organized meal.

We are what we repeatedly do. Excellence, then,
is not an act, but a habit.

—Aristotle

7. Eat earlier

Shift the majority of the calories you consume to earlier in the day and cut out the late-night eating and snacks.

Move dinner up so that you can comfortably stop any intake of calories by 7 p.m. We know that the body tends to hold on to calories consumed late at night and burns calories eaten early in the day. In fact, people who consume the exact same net amount of calories and burn the same amount of calories under controlled settings will actually gain more weight when they eat those calories late in the night and lose more weight when they burn those same calories early in the day.

But there's something about late evening that makes many people want to snack. Maybe the rest of the family has gone to bed. Maybe you're single and that's the time of day you're most relaxed and your willpower is weakest. This is the time cravings can hit hard. Resist them: Nothing good comes from consuming calories so late at night, and none of them are going to be burned when you go off to bed only a little while later.

But sometimes you absolutely want to have something that tastes good. If you've finally given in to temptation, try to only have a bite or two of the food you are craving and leave the rest as a treat for yourself in the morning. Most of the time you won't even want it anymore.

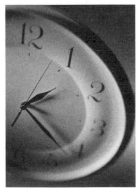

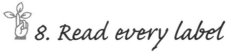

8. Read every label

One of the successful strategies for changing behaviors is a concept called mindfulness. Being mindful can help you change your behavior without outside stimulus (or, perhaps, nagging) by becoming aware or mindful of the consequences of those behaviors. Information leads to insight and a greater appreciation for the consequences of action. As a result, you're much more likely to change your behavior if you're paying attention. It's much harder to indulge in some high-calorie extravagance if you know exactly how many calories are lined up and looking to land in their favorite storage spots on your body.

Knowing the calorie count of everything you buy—and everything you eat—creates mindfulness and limits the high-calorie disasters that can wind up in the refrigerator or on your plate.

Can you become more mindful just by reading a label? Yes. Food labels still leave a lot to be desired, but today there's a set standard to which the FDA expects food manufacturers to conform. So at least the packaging will list calorie content per serving and serving size. There's also generally a breakdown of nutrients, though that can be harder to make sense of because it is not always displayed in a consistent manner.

Nutrition Facts

Serving Size 1 cup (85g) (3 oz.)

Servings per container 2.5

Amount per serving

Calories 45	Calories from Fat 0

	% Daily Value*
Total Fat 0g	0%
Saturated Fat 0g	0%
Cholesterol 0mg	0%
Sodium 55 mg	2%
Total Carbohydrate 10g	3%
Dietary Fiber 3g	12%
Sugars 5g	
Protein 1g	

Vitamin A 360% • Vitamin C 8% • Calcium 2% • Iron 0%

*Percent Daily Values are based on a 2,000 calorie diet. Your daily value may be higher or lower depending on your calorie needs.

	Calories:	2,000	2,500
Total Fat	Less than	65g	80g
Sat. Fat	Less than	20g	25g
Cholesterol	Less than	300mg	300mg
Sodium	Less than	2,400mg	2,400mg
Total Carbohydrate	Less than	300mg	375mg
Dietary Fiber	Less than	25g	30g

Calories per gram: Fat 9 • Carbohydrate 4 • Protein 4

Ingredients: Carrots.

The key here is to read every label, every time. The more familiar you are with reading labels, the more astute you'll become at comparing calorie and carbohydrate contents and really understanding what it is you're eating.

The goal isn't just to reduce calories, but to reduce the carbohydrates you're eating. Read the labels and load the refined sugars into your mental calculator. This doesn't mean you can't eat foods you enjoy—it's more that you need to be aware of what it is you're enjoying. If something is going to add 350 calories to your daily intake, especially if those calories are mostly sugar, whatever it is you're eating better taste very good, because otherwise it's just not worth it.

Remember that food manufacturers play fast and loose with their interpretation of a serving size. They have a vested interest in having you consume their product, so they'll happily tell you there are almost no calories at all in a single serving—and if you don't look too closely you might not notice that a "single serving" consists of a teaspoon's worth. Don't be fooled. Take the time to study the nutritional information, the calorie content and the sugars, and make sure you understand what a serving size is. If you're considering a bag of snacks that's going to take you about three bites to devour, make sure those three bites aren't considered three servings with attendant calorie counts. Food manufacturers can be very sneaky.

Motivation is what gets you started.
Habit is what keeps you going.

—Jim Ryun

9. Plan meals ahead of time

Dinner shouldn't come as a surprise every night. Try planning ahead more than one night at a time ("What should we have for dinner?") and you'll give yourself a chance to find healthier alternatives to fast food, packaged food or the good old standbys like garlic bread and spaghetti. Try to incorporate fresh produce into each planned dinner.

Try writing out a menu for a week at a time. It may be a struggle to get off work and home by 6 or 6:30, or you might have shift work or a busy family with conflicting hours. Planning in advance will help you figure out healthy meals and cut down on prep time (you can prepare ingredients for several nights at a time, slicing, chopping, trimming, soaking, marinating and storing ingredients to use later) and put the family calendar into perspective. If everyone is usually home, alert your family members that you're all going to be eating earlier and do whatever it takes to get home and get cooking on time. If you're not the family chef, have a conversation with whoever does the cooking about eating earlier and offer to help facilitate earlier meals by planning, shopping and helping prepare.

Continuous effort—not strength or intelligence—
is the key to unlocking our potential."

—Liane Cardes

There's a nice side effect to implementing this tip—once you get home earlier, and have shopped and done some of the dinner prep a day or two earlier, you're now going to finish dinner earlier and have more evening time left to do the things you enjoy: taking a walk, spending time with family, reading, watching TV (see Tip 75). Make a new rule: When you watch TV, keep moving, helping the kids with their homework, walking the dog or even writing the great American novel. Who knows what you'll accomplish with that time (other than weight loss)?

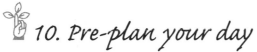

10. Pre-plan your day

Know what you're going to eat, where and when. Just as dinner shouldn't come as a surprise, none of your other food choices should be complete shocks, either. If you're having lunch in a restaurant, consider your order and your substitutions (healthy vs. unhealthy) ahead of time. Figure out how many calories you should reduce at dinner to make up for a restaurant lunch, or how much additional exercise you need to make up for those extra calories. Or for that matter, try to design the most nutritious, low-calorie, low-carb restaurant lunch you can. Make it a contest between you and yourself—one you'll win.

11. Serve yourself on a smaller plate

Most of us are creatures of habit. We're used to using dinner plates for dinner (and maybe breakfast and lunch, too) and we're used to seeing our plates full. Anything else makes us feel we're missing something. But habit can be changed. Serve yourself on a smaller plate and you'll feel just as satisfied.

Meal satisfaction comes from several different components. Taste is important: the differences between salty, savory, sweet and sour. There's a satisfaction to chewing and swallowing. And the first bite of a meal is a pleasure all by itself—how often is the second bite quite as enjoyable?

There's probably also a satisfaction to stuffing ourselves, activating the so-called stretch receptors of the stomach itself (pretty much exactly the sort of pleasure to avoid when seeking to avoid weight gain.) And there seems to be a pleasure in finishing the last bite of a meal.

You can experience most of the same, positive pleasures and satisfactions from a smaller meal, especially when it's packaged on a smaller plate. The first bite, the intense flavors, the last bite. You can still linger over social interaction with dining companions and clean your plate with the psychological satisfaction of a job well-done (or a plate well-cleaned.)

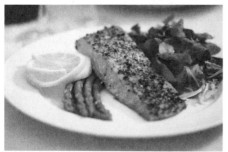

Try serving yourself the same size portions on a smaller plate. Watch to see if your levels of satisfaction don't remain the same and if, over time, your portions don't decrease—though not the pleasure.

12. Leave food on your plate

Make a rule to do the opposite of what your mother told you: Always leave food on your plate. Never finish all of anything, not matter how good it is.

Not to say anything against anyone's mother, but in this case, mother was wrong. She had your best interests at heart, but finishing everything on your plate for the sole purpose of finishing everything on your plate is a bad idea. In today's world of ubiquitous calories and carbohydrates, cleaning your plate means establishing a lifetime habit of weight gain. Especially if you're still using dinner plates (see Tip 11).

 ## 13. Fill your plate only once

Don't have seconds. Leave serving plates on the counter so you have to get up to serve yourself and make it hard to have seconds. After serving up the meal, put the food away: covered, cooled and in the refrigerator. Take your time and enjoy your meal. and when you get up and clear the table, move on immediately to a non-food activity, something maybe more engaging than whatever's on television tonight. It makes it much less likely you'll expend the effort to go back for seconds if you're already doing something else and the food is already put away. Plus putting the food away before sitting down to eat stops you from snacking on leftovers while you're cleaning up.

14. Have dinner and a walk

It's like dinner and a movie, only different. Have a light dinner and take an evening walk. Do this regularly and watch the pounds fall off.

It's amazing how simple changes in behavior can affect not only your weight but your whole life. Taking a walk in the evening, especially when it replaces random snacking and channel surfing, is an excellent way to get fit and lose weight.

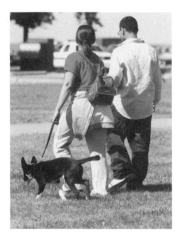

There are collateral benefits, too. Your companion on your walks (even if it's your schnauzer) will enjoy your company, and relationships will be strengthened.

Walking is great exercise. In fact, it's the most sustainable long-term exercise for people who have managed to keep off a significant amount of weight for years. It's good for the mind, body and soul. It gets you out of the house into the fresh air, taking notice of life the way you don't if you stay in the car or the office or on the job site and then watch TV after dinner. There are numerous Web sites that discuss the benefits of walking (I recommend those listed in Appendix E).

 ## 15. Skip dessert in favor of that walk

OK, the first choice many of us make is to finish dinner and watch some TV. Maybe a movie. Or maybe read a book. None of these are as good for your body as a walk.

It might be hard to take that first step out the front door, but eventually you'll wonder how you ever lived without those after-dinner walks. When you get back, have a big glass of ice water instead of diving into the calories. Tell yourself you're skipping dessert tonight.

Dessert should be a special treat, not a routine occurrence. If you're already overweight and trying to move back to a healthy weight, there's even less rationale for eating dessert on a regular basis. Start skipping it. Take that walk instead. And if dessert makes its way back onto the menu every now and then, it will have become a treat. At my house, instead of asking, "What's for dessert?" my kids ask, "Is tonight a dessert night?"

16. Brush your teeth an hour earlier

After dinner, when it's time for your walk, or time to read or watch TV, about the time you change into your sweats or your pajamas and get comfortable, take a minute and brush your teeth. Who doesn't like to have fresh, minty, clean teeth?

Once you've brushed your teeth, have nothing but ice water for the rest of the night. This simple step can help you avoid taking in needless, mindless calories by snacking on popcorn or trail mix, sweets or salty things that many of us crave in the evening. Most of the time we don't need these calories; we're not really hungry; we're just watching TV or reading a book. Since these late-night calories are the most likely to be immediately deposited and stored as fat, they're some of the most important calories to avoid.

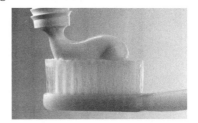

17. Get enough sleep

Studies show millions of people in this country are suffering from chronic sleep deprivation. Studies also show that sleep deprivation has a direct impact on weight gain (Patel, 2006) and that we eat more and metabolize less with sleep deprivation.

Human beings need seven to eight hours of sleep a night, and it's become harder and harder to get that. Put together the stress of the job, the hours with the kids, the household duties, the worry about the economy and the escalating price of gas, plus all the electronic ways in which our jobs can go on long past the hours actually spent at the work site, and it's no wonder so many of us aren't sleeping.

You may find it hard to turn off your thoughts and fall asleep, or you may find yourself waking up after a few hours unable to return to sleep. Depression and stress can both cause you to wake during the night and stay awake. If this is what's keeping you from getting your Zs you may be able to solve the problem with a visit to your doctor, or you may look to a more complicated answer involving a diagnostic sleep study or counseling.

Keep away from people who try to belittle your ambitions. Small people always do that, but the really great make you feel that you, too, can become great.

—Mark Twain

There are also physical reasons you may not be sleeping well. Chronic pain can interrupt sleep. Many people who are overweight suffer from a medical sleep disturbance such as sleep apnea. If you know that you snore or anyone has ever told you that you snore (and people are often likely to tell you the minute your snoring wakes them) you may have sleep apnea. Another symptom is a temporary pause in breathing. Stopping breathing or ongoing snoring are both major signs that you have sleep apnea that needs to be treated.

Sleep deprivation means more than just being groggy in the morning. Along with the actual physical stresses to the body, sleep deprivation hurts your chances of losing weight. And just as importantly, losing weight will help you sleep better. Talk to your doctor. Ask about sleep studies and potential psychological or stress-related causes to your sleep impairment. If you live with someone who can witness your sleep habits, find out if that person has noticed anything unusual. Get professional help if you need it—it's important.

Set your goals high and don't stop until you get there.

—Bo Jackson

The Goal: Setting Goals

18. Play defense

Most of the time it isn't the burst of intensive workouts that produces the great weight-loss results in the long run, it's the small, short-term, repeated efforts that win the day. While a 10-mile run may be exhilarating, it's not likely to be the key that leads to long-term weight loss. Instead, it's the small, determined and sustained effort to keep high-carb snacks and foods out of the grocery cart and out of the pantry—day after day after day—that makes the difference.

Call it a good day when you succeed at playing defense by avoiding the onslaught of fast food lures and food advertising, when you skip dessert and avoid the temptations at the office candy bowl or doughnut buffet. Maybe you didn't run a marathon today or bench press more than your body weight but you played good defense. You strengthened your commitment to weight loss and your habits of eating healthier and lowering the calorie and carb consumption. That's a good day.

Playing defense is not always flashy or sexy; but it wins games. In this case, the game is your long-term health, and the stakes couldn't be higher.

When I work in the medical setting with patients who need to lose weight, I find it very valuable to set clear, well-defined goals. This means that in addition to a specific number of pounds they want to lose within a specific time frame, they also need to think about the specific reasons they want to lose those pounds.

Losing weight is like a long-term project that requires a detailed blueprint. You need to create your blueprint carefully and look at it daily. With a solid blueprint, you have a strong, mapped-out approach to your project and a much better chance of succeeding at attaining a healthier weight, feeling better and living longer.

19. List your top five reasons for losing weight

Write down the following: The top five reasons I want to lose weight are…List the reasons in order. Read the list. Every day.

There's something powerful and tangible about writing down your reasons and identifying your goals. You may already know all the reasons you want to lose weight but writing them down clarifies your intentions. It's one thing to know you feel better at a specific weight and another to identify and write down that your passion is cross-country skiing and you want to go back to it. Take your time with this goal. It's important to understand why you're embarking on the weight-loss journey.

Here are a few number-one goals from my patients:

⬦ I want to ride horses with my granddaughter.
⬦ I want to wear my favorite jeans and have them look good on me.
⬦ I want to stop taking blood pressure medication and have normal blood pressure.

◇ I want to sleep the whole night through without waking up, and then I want to wake up feeling rested in the morning.

◇ I want to end the day without my back or knees or hips hurting.

There are so many pleasures in life that make it wonderful to be alive, and so many favorite things become harder to do or less enjoyable with weight gain. One of my patients told me he dropped his car keys and spent an embar- 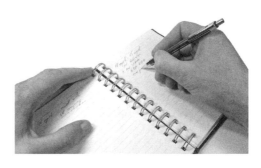 rassing 15 minutes trying to bend down safely to pick them up. Ten years ago, in his 40s and probably 50 pounds overweight, he'd never imagined he'd go through something like that. But the extra pounds and extra years and a bad knee made bending down to pick up keys a serious and tricky proposition. His number-one goal on his Top Five list? To be able to bend down and pick up his keys easily without falling and without getting hurt.

Alter your attitude and you will change your life.

—William Arthur Ward

20. Post your reasons

Write your list of reasons to lose weight on a sticky note or index card and stick it somewhere you'll see it—on the refrigerator or the bathroom mirror. Make several copies, even, and post them where they will inspire you—in the car, in a desk drawer you open every day, in your gym bag.

21. Make realistic goals

When you're making a list of goals for weight loss, it's easy to get excited by the prospect and make unrealistic goals. It's possible to be diligent and take steps to lose weight quickly, but it's still going to take some time and unrealistic goals that you can't meet can make it feel like you're failing when you're actually succeeding (if you're losing the weight, you're succeeding!)

Be patient, and don't give up. You should try to lose between one and two pounds a week initially, then even less per week after the first six months. Shedding even 10 pounds of excess weight has been shown to have significant health benefits. Once you've lost 10 pounds, set out to lose another 10.

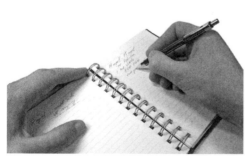

22. Tell your friends

Communicate your needs and plans to friends and family. Ask for support and understanding as you make your journey toward improved health. Understand that some people are going to be threatened by the changes you're making. You're becoming a new person, and some people aren't ready to give up the person you used to be.

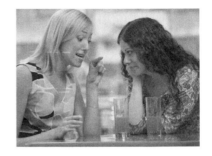

Watch for saboteurs. Sabotage can come from expected quarters, like bad habits (the daily soda, the popcorn or chips with a favorite daily or weekly television show, the nightly dessert) but can also come from unexpected sources such as otherwise supportive friends who seem unwilling to understand that meeting in the same place at the same time ignites the same expectations of the same treats as have always been shared. And some friends will resent losing a pal they've always eaten with.

Align yourself with those people in your life who will be most supportive. Successful weight-loss programs are something like successful friendships: They take a lot of work and love and commitment, understanding and perseverance. Start yours off with a public celebration that invites support and brings out the best in everyone around you. Announce your excitement at the changes you're planning and ask others to join in your pleasure. Don't keep it a secret!

23. Blog it

In the brave new world of online journals you can find someone to share any passion you can dream up—including weight loss. From professional bloggers (see my blog on weight loss at www. sasseguide.com/blog/sasse-guide-blog/) to those people jogging along the same weight-loss path you're on, there's plenty of company. There are even weight-loss tracking software programs that can be downloaded to blogs, computers and phones that will chart your progress as your bathroom scale tips ever lower. A quick Google of weight-loss tracking software will give you many options and stay tuned for an upcoming weight-loss tracking module on the iMetabolic.com Web site. If you'd like company on your journey you may be able to find an entire community of people to support you on your way.

24. Join a support group

Talk to others about your weight-loss goals. Studies show that participation in support groups improves weight-loss success (Levy, 1993). It makes sense. People are social creatures who involve others in the highs and lows of life. We celebrate with

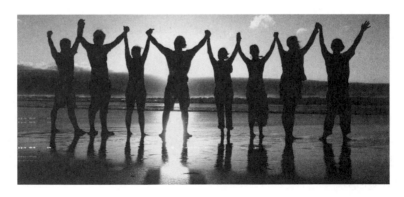

others. We call friends when we're down. And many of our social interactions revolve around food. It's nice to go to a social event that doesn't. Not only that, but when a project is tricky, we ask other people for advice.

Losing weight is difficult. Keeping it off long-term is difficult. Everyone has those low willpower moments or times when we're depressed or sad or anxious or just plain bored and we want to eat. So it makes sense it might help to get together in a group and talk—what works, what doesn't, what triggers us to overeat. The task of losing weight becomes easier when you've got a group of like-minded friends supporting you. They can help you through low moments and celebrate the high moments.

25. Find a supportive friend

If groups don't work for you—or if you'd like additional backup for those moments when willpower has waned and temptation grown—call a friend or support person before you binge on something terrible. You are important to the people who love you, so your goals for improved health and long-term weight loss are important to them, too.

We all have those moments of backsliding, forgetting, eating mindlessly without paying attention. A moment like that can happen at any time: You can have an amazing month of eating right and working out and lose your momentum in one binge. From there, it's an easy step to the next backslide or to giving up altogether.

Don't let this happen. Line up a friend or two or three—anyone you know who is hardcore in your camp, cheering you on. Ask if these friends are willing to be your support system, and when they say yes and you feel that willpower start to flicker, call them.

A friend's concerned and thoughtful responses could stand between you and a relapse that causes you to regain the weight you've lost.

26. Be your own cheerleader

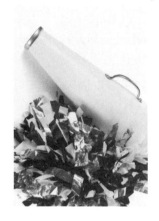

Love yourself. Decide to lose the excess weight because you're wonderful and you deserve it. Remind yourself you're already a unique and special person, not planning to become one. Make the changes and lose the weight to improve your own health for your own sake. Don't wait until you hit your goal weight to do something nice for yourself. Make a list of non-food rewards for reaching milestone weights.

27. Substitute good habits in place of bad habits

Habits can't be broken, only changed. So, rather than trying to quit a learned behavior cold turkey, substitute a new, healthy alternative. Rather than trying to break bad habits, chip away at them. Rather than making sweeping changes to every sector of your life, start with small, easily achieved changes. If you can't go through the day without chocolate, rather than trying to completely give up something you love and ending up binging or making yourself miserable only to fall off the wagon, make a substitution. Rather than a 650-calorie piece of cake, try a 100-calorie dark chocolate bar with its attendant antioxidants and health benefits. You'll be replacing a lot of sugar and fat and still enjoying the taste you love.

Change bad habits to more acceptable habits geared toward long-term weight-loss success. And don't give up—these changes aren't going to happen overnight but only through repetition, repetition, repetition until the new behaviors are ingrained and feel natural.

The temptation to slip back into old behaviors is natural and can take a year or longer to fade away. Substituting new, healthy habits for old, unhealthy habits makes learning new behaviors easier.

28. Surround yourself with friends who have met their weight goals

Weight loss—and weight gain—are contagious. Maybe not contagious in the medical sense of the word. But studies have shown that if your friends are successfully losing weight or they are normal weight or healthy, fit people, your odds of becoming healthier and more fit, and losing weight and maintaining that weight loss, are better.

I'm not suggesting you lose every friend who doesn't conform to a certain clothing size, or that you go out of your way to cultivate the friendships of the very skinny. If your friends arc overweight as well, you may be the catalyst to change that. Tell your friends about your weight-loss plans. Invite them to join you. Enlist their aid and support and offer them yours. If you're all moving in the same direction, toward fitness and weight loss, you've all got a much better chance of achieving your goals of better health, better quality of life, longer life and a smaller waistline.

29. Weigh yourself every day

Studies show to lose weight, we are most successful when we weigh ourselves daily and keep focused on our goals. Personally, I fought this one for a while, but eventually the data won me over. In this weight-obsessed culture and the body-image-focused media, I'm cautious about making a blanket recommendation that everyone focus every day on their weight. But when discussing the increasing majority of people who need to lose weight, this becomes more of a health issue than a cultural or social issue.

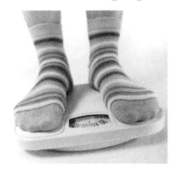

For people who are overweight and trying to lose that weight, the focus needs to be on exercise, nutrition and pounds lost. So, if you're trying to lose pounds, then you need to keep track of your weight, and weighing daily or at least several times a week is part of that effort, just like counting carbohydrates and paying attention to everything you eat.

30. Find out what you're made of

Learn the truth about your body fat percentage so you can reduce it if you need to. Test your body composition at a weight-loss center or health club. Or, if you want to find out what your body fat percentage is without leaving home and involving someone else in the computations, try the "home body fat test" for a rough estimate (http://www.healthcentral.com/cholesterol/home-body-fat-test-2774-143.html) or check out the Body Mass Index in Appendix C.

Body composition analyzers have become extremely accurate at measuring the percentages of lean body mass and fat mass. A normal body fat percentage is 10 to 20 percent for men and generally 18 to 28 percent for women. (See Figure 1.) You should know your percentage of body fat and make an effort to reduce it if it's over the limit.

Body fat is more than just a place for the storage of extra calories. It's actually increasingly thought to be an important endocrine organ, a body part that makes hormones (special chemicals in the bloodstream that send out signals to control the metabolism). Fat stores are an organ of the body spread out the way skin is spread out, which means fat should be thought of as an organ distributed in various places throughout the

Exercise has categorized ranges of body fat percentages as follows:

Description	Women	Men
Essential fat	12-15%	2-5%
Athletes	16-29%	6-13%
Fitness	21-24%	14-17%
Acceptable	25-31%	18-25%
Obese	32%+	25%+

[Reference : http://www.healthchecksystems.com/bodyfat.htm]

body. The fat cells work together to secrete potent hormones that affect our bodies' regulatory systems (Kissebah, 1982). Increasing the activity of these fat stores leads to reduced insulin sensitivity. Reduced insulin sensitivity is a precursor of diabetes.

Figure 1—Normal Body Fat Percentage for the average population of the U.S. and Western World: *Today, people are exhibiting higher percentages of body fat than shown, a very unhealthy trend.*

Body Fat Percentage for the average population.			
Age	**Up to 30**	**30 to 50**	**50+**
Females	14-21%	15-23%	16-25%
Males	9-15%	11-17%	12-19%

[The best way to lose weight is to reduce intake of calories and carbohydrates, and increase exercise to burn off the fat. The key is to reduce the body fat percentage and maintain or preserve the lean body mass or muscle mass. Maintaining lean muscle while losing excess body fat will lead to less rebound weight gain (Sasse, 2008).]

31. Bad days happen to everyone

Don't collapse, don't throw in the towel; don't give up. Relapses happen to everyone, so just refocus and restart. Just because you had a bad day and ate something you shouldn't have or celebrated an event the wrong, food-related, way doesn't make you a bad person. It makes you human. Making changes to your behavior is difficult. Smokers often quit eight to 12 times before they kick the habit for good. Is this a fair comparison? Pretty much. Though smokers can certainly live without smoking and none of us can live without food, giving up junk food—the stuff we don't need, that doesn't sustain life—is a lot like giving up smoking. Successful weight loss takes perseverance and self-control and the willingness to try, try again.

Sometimes you're going to have a relapse into old, bad food habits. Sometimes you'll even lose ground and regain weight you've lost. You're human. It happens. Move on.

The key is to gather yourself, refocus your intentions, restate your goals and restart. Remind yourself what your goals are and why you want to achieve them. Pull out your list of important reasons for losing weight and review it. Call your support group or support friends. Any time you make an important decision and try to change something for the best, your resolve will be tempted. Don't judge; don't condemn yourself.

Commit yourself to making lifelong changes in behavior in order to sustain long-term weight loss. One or two lapses in judgment don't constitute failure. Giving up does. You can do it. You can succeed. Never giving up is at the core of long-term success.

Medically-supervised weight-loss programs can bring a higher level of sophistication and higher level of success to your weight-loss journey. This section of the book will explore many of the root causes of weight gain and ideas for how to fight back.

Many of us spend time taking care of others and worrying about our needs last. In this section we'll take a look at changes you can make just for yourself. In many cases no one else even needs to know about them. And when you start celebrating your success at weight loss, you'll know who to thank. Good for you!

32. Start a food log

Keep an accurate record of everything you eat for a week. Don't judge; just record, accurately. Studies show it is easier to lose weight with the aid of a record of everything eaten.

There are obviously plenty of reasons why food logs work, but chief among them is that recording everything creates mindfulness. If you keep a log, it forces you to maintain a much higher level of awareness of the food and drink you're consuming. It's a lot harder to cheat when everything you ate during the day is right there in black and white. It makes it harder to forget or deny that doughnut or the croissant that slipped by your defenses. It's also harder to actually do the cheating when you realize after you get done enjoying your brief indulgence you're going to have to write down the details. You may choose to forgo your dubious pleasure.

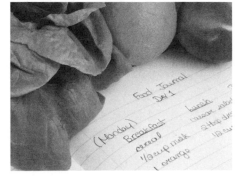

In the beginning, record absolutely everything you eat, no matter how seemingly insignificant or how small. A few chips or a handful of popcorn at work might seem insignificant, but it adds up over the course of the day or the week. Write down everything, even the healthy stuff, the vegetables and fruits and the things you only took one bite of. As time goes on you'll probably find your own shorthand method of taking notes, but at the beginning, write everything down. You may want to include the calorie count, as well. And if you want to break it down further and get an idea what you're really eating, separate out the calories from carbohydrates, fats and protein.

Don't make value judgments. Don't make changes to your behavior. Don't try to focus on reducing or eliminating what you're eating just because you're going to write it down. Just focus on faithfully recording everything. Right now you're just trying to understand everything you eat, when and where. In time, this heightened awareness and mindfulness will lead to inevitable changes in your eating habits, but don't worry about that in the beginning. Just learn to observe, record and be mindful.

33. Be honest with yourself

Don't bother cheating or omitting things when you're keeping a food log. For one thing, the person you're answering to is yourself, and you already know what you're trying to hide. The truth, in this instance, will definitely win out.

Keeping an honest daily food log will help you determine the times of day and in what situations you're most likely to lose control over your food choices, and develop an effective "battle plan" you can stick with. More than likely you're the only person who is ever going to read your food log, so use it for your goals list, your journal-keeping and your weigh-ins as well as tracking your food intake within its pages. Don't bother telling lies. Write down the bitter truth, no matter how embarrassing.

34. Keep a record of the calories you *don't* eat

Did you skip the doughnut in the conference room at work this morning? Good for you! Award yourself 250 calories. Did you request your potatoes without gravy? You've just saved 150 calories. At the end of the day when totaling up your food log, take a look at how many calories you *almost* ate but didn't. Then reward yourself, but not with food and especially not with food at the end of the day. Instead, find a way to reward yourself for the calories you *didn't* eat. Start saving up calories and "spend" them

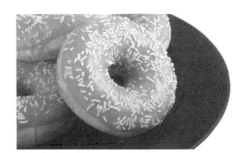

on a new pair of shoes. Or a massage. Or a fishing trip. It feels good to narrowly escape the clutches of hundreds of calories a day, so take note of these small victories on your path to a healthy weight.

35. Clean the pantry

Pick a day to go through on a systematic search-and-destroy mission and clean out the pantry and the cupboards and the refrigerator of all the junk food. Get it out of the house. If it's not there, you can't eat it. If you can't stand to throw it away, give it away, preferably not to someone else trying to lose weight, but, really, the world will go on even if you throw out that half-eaten package of Oreos.

Note of caution: Do not attempt this when you are very hungry.

Is this a tough assignment? You bet. The key is admitting we all have our ups and downs when it comes to willpower. Do your best to fend off that moment when you're not stronger than your favorite junk food. The fact that some day you may not be stronger than your favorite snacks doesn't mean you'll have failed—throwing it out in a preemptive strike means you're winning.

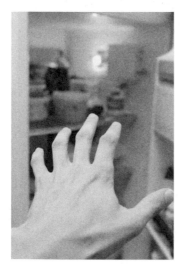

So root it out and throw it out. Put it down the disposal. Throw it in the trash with the chicken skins and onion peels. Do whatever it takes to make sure it isn't going to come back and take up residence in your pantry again.

When your willpower is down and you're tired and sore and cranky from the workout you just had (good for you!) and the need for something *really bad* strikes you, the bad stuff won't be there. I know. I've done this myself. I've made sure my home and office are safe from my favorite chocolates and snacks. By doing this you can save yourself a bunch of calories and a bunch of new pounds. You'll probably even lose some.

And, sure, there might come a day when you really mean business and you think about going to pick up your keys and head for the nearest convenience store. I've been there, too. Most of the time, it's just too darn much work. Which is a good thing.

The tragedy in life doesn't lie in not reaching your goal.
The tragedy lies in having no goal to reach.

—Benjamin Mays

36. Ban trans fats

Root out the unhealthy snacks in your pantry and any prepared foods that might be harboring trans fats and get rid of them. And don't bring any more in. Read labels. Make sure. Take it from the American Heart Association: These are bad for you.

Trans fats are finally being acknowledged as harmful to human health. It's taken awhile to get here, but now everyone from health authorities to the U.S. government agree trans fats have no role in the human diet. These fats are deadly. They congeal and promote plaque deposits in our arteries, leading to heart attacks and strokes and a host of medical problems (Hu, 1997 & Hu, 2002). Health authorities have reduced the recommended allowance of trans fasts in the human diet to exactly zero. (For more information on trans fat, please visit the U.S. Food and Drug Administration site: http://www.cfsan. fda.gov/~dms/qatrans2.html.)

37. Find an empathetic and caring bariatric physician

Weight management is a very difficult endeavor. It's made even harder when you try to go it alone. A skilled, caring physician in your corner can boost your chances of short-term and long-term success. Physicians trained in the bariatric field are your best hope of finding safe and effective medical weight-loss care.

One way to find a bariatric physician is through the American Society of Bariatric Physicians, the professional organization for physicians specializing in medically-supervised weight loss. Visit www.asbp.org to find a weight-loss specialist where you live. In addition, many doctors have developed a specialty in the field of weight loss through their extensive experience in bariatric surgery, endocrinology, internal medicine or other fields.

Most of these doctors have a medically-supervised plan you can begin right away. And with medical supervision, you can lose weight safely and stay on top of those other health conditions that need attention.

38. Use a pedometer

Buy a pedometer. Wear it daily. Keep track of the number of steps you're walking every day.

At Western Bariatric Institute, we started giving out pedometers to patients and staff alike. The enthusiasm was contagious, and, in no time, people were competing against each other, checking in to see who had done how many steps the day before, competing to do more the next day.

Use a pedometer to count the number of steps you take every day. Set a goal for a minimum number of steps. Once you've started achieving your goal you'll find you're ready to push further. You'll find yourself parking farther away from where you're going and taking the stairs rather than the elevator just so you can count more steps. Good for you! This is a behavioral change for the better. When you're trying to hit a goal every day, you feel better; when you hit or exceed that goal, you feel better still. And instead of letting your mind drift and find ways of being lazier—shortcuts and escalators and driving from one store in the same parking lot to the next—your brain is working competitively, adding steps, beating goals.

There are a lot of models of pedometers out there. I recommend starting with a simple version. If you end up hooked (and you hopefully will) you can always upgrade to a fancy pedometer that will help you convert the length of your stride into mileage and perform other functions such as operating like a stopwatch.

39. Take at least 8,000 steps a day

No, you're probably not looking to train for a marathon or even a 5K. At least not yet. You don't have to jump from 5,000 to 12,000 steps in a day or even a week. In fact, most trainers suggest not increasing workouts by more than 10 percent a week. So if you started with 8,000, you'd increase to 8,800 (but you might as well shoot for 9,000, right?). And once you're used to one level, moving up 10 percent doesn't require that much more effort. What it *does* do is dramatically increase your long-term weight loss success.

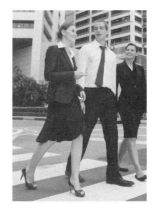

It takes around 2,000 steps to equal one mile of walking, give or take, depending on the length of your stride. So recording 8,000 steps in your day means you've walked around four miles. Pretty good. For many people who have gained weight over the past years, and have fairly sedentary jobs, this goal is a good one to shoot for.

40. Learn to live with some hunger

That doesn't sound good, does it? But hunger is no longer the evolution-fueled drive it once was. Let's face it, you're not going out and hunting down a wooly mammoth for dinner. In fact, in many instances, you don't have to raise more than a finger and dinner is summoned to your front door. And therein lies the problem.

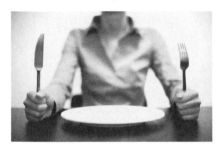

We live in a modern society, but we still have caveman genes. Scientists believe that early man lived in hunter-gatherer tribes, with diets that consisted of small prey they could trap fairly often, large prey that took more work and was achieved less frequently and natural fruits that were obtainable at various times of the year. With such a diet, early man had to live with some hunger probably most of the time, and what's more, had to work to procure dinner by chasing it and killing it, effectively working off the calories before ever consuming them.

Today we don't have these challenges. Woolly mammoths would be protected if they were still around and it takes hardly any calories at all to get the keys and drive to the drive-through where the only thing limiting the amount of food you can get is the size of your wallet. Easier still, many restaurants deliver, right to your front door. Lift a finger, burn half a calorie, order 30 pizzas. It's not a healthy equation.

Hunger served humans well when we had to plan and stalk and kill our food in order to consume calories. Hunger doesn't serve us so well in today's society when we're surrounded by bad food choices, all instantly available.

You need to think of hunger differently. Stop thinking of hunger as a need that must be met. I'll say this again, because it's an important concept and one that's difficult to grasp, but: If you live in the U.S. or any technologically advanced civilization where food is readily available, you need to stop thinking about hunger being a need that must be met. It is no longer a beneficial impulse to answer the needs of hunger. If you are overweight, hunger is harmful, destructive to your life, not helpful.

Remember that each gram of protein or carbohydrate contains four calories, and each gram of fat contains nine. And each gram of carbohydrates flows directly into the bloodstream and raises the blood glucose level and triggers the surges of hormones associated with obesity.

So a bar that has 15 grams of protein already has 60 calories. Add in 10 grams of carbohydrates (40 calories) and your total is now 100 calories. Another 100 calories from fat (11 grams of fat) and you've got a 200 calorie protein bar.

So beware a bar that lists 30 grams of sugar—that bar already has 120 calories without adding in the protein and fat and is going to cause too rapid a rise in blood sugar.

Hunger is not something to be listened to, accommodated or responded to at its every whim. Instead, hunger is something that must be controlled, lived with and, in some cases, outright ignored. Hunger is a sign that you've cut unnecessary calories. When you experience hunger you're in a period of weight loss. If you don't give in and eat, the body is forced to look to stores of fat for energy. Look on hunger pangs and a growling stomach as a sign of weight loss. The control you develop here may be your greatest asset in weight loss.

If you haven't lived with hunger, this may seem intolerable, but try it. Try not assuaging your hunger in the evening. See what it feels like. Take stock of your body and mind. It won't hurt you to be hungry briefly. It won't result in injury or illness to your body or mind, organs or bones or any part of your system. Strangely enough, it will soon feel natural and even comfortable to live with some hunger.

One last note: Every overweight person I've helped who has mastered this point of learning to live with hunger tells me that even though it's hard to adjust to at first, it feels infinitely better to live with some hunger than to be overweight.

Want a ballpark of how many calories a day you need in your daily life or daily grind? Or an idea of a baseline calorie count to start subtracting from in order to lose weight? Try the calorie counter at http://hubpages.com/hub/How_To_Calculate_Your_Calorie_Needs

41. Practice eating until you're satisfied, not full

There's a difference between feeling full and feeling satisfied—a difference of probably several hundred calories a day.

Feeling full means feeling that you've eaten too much. It's pushing yourself away from the table declaring "I couldn't eat another bite!" and being right. Being full teeters on the edge of being nauseated. Legend has it that the gluttonous ancient Romans used to feast until they vomited, then started over again. In today's world eating like an ancient Roman would be considered gauche and downright disgusting, let alone remarkably unhealthy.

Feeling satisfied is not the same as feeling full. It means you've eaten what you need to fuel yourself. You've replaced the calories you've burned since you last ate and provided yourself with enough fuel to go do whatever's next.

But how do you know when you've had enough? It takes some trial and error. Most people could probably stop sooner than they do. It becomes a question of choice, taste and enjoyment rather than need. It takes willpower and practice, but if you experiment for a while, you can find a modest portion that will fill you up enough and let you go on with your activities feeling satisfied. The trick is to find the lower limit so that you're satisfied and don't feel the need for dessert or to finish everything on your plate or to start snacking again right after your meal.

When you should stop depends on your body size and body weight. It depends on what we call lean body mass (or muscle mass). It depends on your resting metabolic rate, the number of daily calories burned by your body, which is dependent on lean body mass. But suffice it to say, most people today should stop sooner rather than later, and sooner than they currently do.

For example, suppose you're a woman with a resting metabolic rate of 1,300 calories a day (a qualified bariatric physician can test this for you). That means for a normal day you need 1,300 calories just to get through it.

Here are some rough guidelines for someone who has a resting metabolic rate of 1,300 calories a day (a pretty common rate for someone who is overweight): For breakfast, try a protein bar, preferably one in the 200-calorie range with about 15 grams of protein. There are a number of commercial bars that are good (see Appendix F). Read the label of any bar you're considering—some are unhealthy choices with high fat or high carbohydrate contents or just plain too many calories. For lunch, try half a sandwich with whole grain bread, lean meat, lettuce and tomato and a small amount of low fat or nonfat mayonnaise. For dinner consider four or five ounces of lean chicken and a cup-sized serving of vegetables.

For someone in a physically demanding job, with a basal metabolic rate in the neighborhood of 1,700 calories a day, try adding an egg to that breakfast, an additional ounce or so of the lean lunch meat, maybe lean ground beef or canned tuna. Dinner might include more of the lean chicken and vegetables. But breakfast, even for someone with a demanding, on-your-feet job, isn't going to include juice, toast or a bagel—all that gets you is one-way ticket to obesity and diabetes.

Take a look at the servings in the examples above. Most likely they're smaller than what you normally consume. But that's the point—the servings recommended here are satisfying but not filling and are enough to fuel a body to get on with the day while still resulting in weight loss. This isn't the kind of change to be made overnight, rather, it's something to be approached gradually. Work toward these kinds of quantities. Practice consuming smaller quantities and see how it feels.

42. Slow down

Take plenty of time to talk when eating. Enjoy the conversation and the social aspect of your meal. If you run out of time and you've done more talking than eating, great! If you eat a majority of your meals alone, read a good book while you eat, or look at catalogs featuring equipment for sports you want to try after you lose weight or places you want to visit. Pause and enjoy your food and make your meal an enjoyable experience, but don't get so caught up in what you're reading that you go on nibbling and reading after you've finished your meal.

Multitasking and speed are the orders of the day. You're expected to do more than one thing at a time and you're expected to do them quickly and these expectations don't stop at meals. You *can* stop them, though. Enjoy your meal as a chance to sit down without doing anything other than eating and talking with friends. Don't work; don't worry; don't even watch TV. Think about what you're eating and make it last. Chew each bite thoroughly, 30 times, and experience the tastes and textures of the food. Set aside time for your meal rather than cramming it between more events.

And don't worry—if you don't finish in time, you'll survive. (Even if you do have time to finish, relax—no one is going to rush in and take your plate away. Eat as much as you want.)

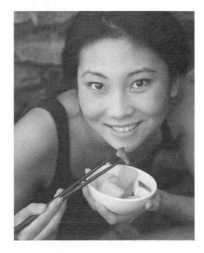

In fact, in the beginning, while you're learning to relax and enjoy your food, don't worry about portion control or whether or not you're finishing.

Just concentrate on going slowly. After you've tried this a few times you can start considering how much you eat, and by then you'll probably have realized you can leave the last third of the meal on the plate.

If you've taken the time to let the food settle, you're more likely to feel satisfied. If you get up from the table and still feel a little bit hungry, give yourself 20 minutes. Often at the end of that time you'll find your body has caught up to what's been happening and you're now satisfied with the food you've eaten.

The chains of habit are generally too small to be felt until they are too strong to be broken.

—Samuel Johnson

43. Are you ready for some football

Football itself has very few calories. Football food is another story. And then there's beer—carbs in a bottle. I'm not going to assume you're never going to indulge again, but there's a way to get from Saturday to Monday and enjoy the game in the process without gaining back everything you've lost. If, for you, beer and football go together like snowfall and Christmas, first try a lower carb, lower calorie beer, and second, for every beer, have a full glass of ice water. You'll cut down on the number of beers you drink throughout the game, and as a bonus, reduce your chances of a hangover.

Giving up the football food, all those chips and dips, might seem painful, but start putting out trays of fresh carrots and celery. The game won't be any less exciting and you'll enjoy it just as much, plus you'll still have crunchy foods to go with all the action.

Medical weight loss knowledge has come a long way. Today we can point to sophisticated research on many types of foods and advise patients on what is truly healthy, and what isn't. For people seeking to lose weight and become healthier, there are many, many important points about specific dietary choices that should be known.

Many of these tips run counter to what the commercial food industry would have people believe. The medical weight-loss specialty does not have anywhere near as large a megaphone as the commercial food supply industry, so it stands to reason that many of these pieces of information have escaped public notice.

It's a dream until you write it down,
and then its a goal.

—Anonymous

Never, never, never, never give up.

—Winston Churchill

Fueling and Refueling: Food

Below are the most valuable tips on specific foods and diets that I give to my weight-loss patients. The more of these you can incorporate into your own personal weight-loss plan, the healthier you will be.

44. Learn about a sensible, well-balanced diet

A sensible, well-balanced diet includes a wide variety of whole grains, lean meats and fresh fruits and vegetables. Restrict your consumption of sugars first and foremost, followed by fat.

Believe it or not, the concept of a "healthy diet" still raises controversy. Many experts have, for years, emphasized the idea of low-fat, because, they reasoned, fat has the most calories per gram or per serving. But low-carb is quickly becoming a major contender. For resources and more information on eating well and following the best diet possible, see Appendix F.

45. Make food cuts that don't hurt

Find some carbohydrates in your life that you can live without and then do so. If there are foods that you eat on a daily basis that have just become rote, that don't bring you pleasure or nutrition but do bring you unwelcome calories, it's time to root them out of your diet.

It occurred to me one day that I really don't love potatoes all that much. I like them, sure, and French fries are absolutely heavenly, fresh, hot and salty. But the more I learned about carbohydrates and the more mindful I became of what I was eating, the more I realized I could never do without the occasional chocolate, but I really could live without potatoes. So, potatoes became one thing I can easily skip when they're on my plate. Many restaurant meals come with potatoes; I just don't bother

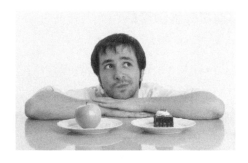

eating them. Crazy as it seems, once you start this type of thing you will actually look forward to having a big potato (or whatever your chosen "leave behind" items are) appear as a side-dish, because you know you will get full credit for not touching any of those particular carbs. And for me, at least, cutting out almost all potatoes has been painless. There is probably some big-carb food that would be painless for you to cut out, too.

You don't have to have fries with that and you don't have to finish the whole packet if you do choose them.

If you've gotten to the end of a meal and been physically satisfied but emotionally unfulfilled, those are probably some extra calories you could do without. This doesn't mean you should throw out the healthy choices like broccoli just because they're not your favorite vegetable. It means if you're not in love with something but eat it out of habit, stop. This may be the sesame seed buns wrapped around the all-beef patties. No one says you can't deconstruct your hamburger—American advertising guarantees you can have it your way and getting rid of the bun disposes of a lot of white flour and simple carbohydrate calories.

You don't even have to eat every meal just because you've been conditioned to. While breakfast is a good idea (a healthy breakfast will help you rev up your metabolism and burn more calories all day), if lunch leaves you feeling limp for hours afterward while you digest and you'd rather have an apple or a handful of nuts or a protein shake, go ahead. If you're not hungry at lunch and ravenous at dinner, try eating a combination meal earlier. You'll have the advantage of missing that post-lunch sag and the added advantage of eating dinner early and skipping late-night calories.

Make simple, painless cuts in your food intake, starting with something you don't like that much and won't miss, and the process of elimination will be much simpler. It's easy once you get used to it, and it feels good, too. Don't eat things just because they're there. Eat foods that count and are delicious, satisfying and healthy.

46. Try fresh game and cold water fish for your main course

Lean meats are excellent natural sources of protein, omega-3 fatty acids and healthy vitamins and minerals. Fresh game and cold water fish are lean meats. They are just plain good for you because the less processed food is, the less preserved, the less hormone-fed, the less synthetic, the better it is for your body.

For most people, today's diet has moved sharply away from the fresh foods, meats and vegetables that are the healthiest choices, including grains, berries, cold water fish and fresh

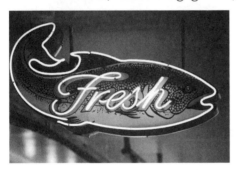

game. Some researchers suggest these foods in particular are the best foods we could eat and that our health has suffered and weight increased, as a population, as a result of shifting away from meals that include these foods.

47. Spice it up

Eating spicy hot peppers in your meals has been shown to increase caloric consumption by the body during the digestive process (Yoshioka, 1999). If you're looking for a spicy recipe to give this a try, take a look at Chef Dave Fouts' Tex-Mex Turkey Chili in Appendix A. Guaranteed spicy.

48. Do a mini-fast

A miniature fast is nowhere near as intimidating as something Ghandi might embark upon. It isn't difficult, and it isn't permanent: Just stop eating after 6 p.m. and don't start up again until somewhere between 6 and 8 a.m. the following day. Studies show this burns fat and lowers insulin. You can repeat the mini-fast three times a week if it works for you.

One unexpected aspect to this particular tip is that you'll actually start to look forward to it. Sound unlikely? It happens.

And a mini-fast can happen unexpectedly. Do you ever forget to eat lunch? Instead of getting caught up, consider eating an early satisfying-but-simple supper around 5 p.m. and then knocking off the food for the night. You've just solved the age-old question about what to do about dinner—nothing! You're done for the night after a simple supper.

Most people who try a mini-fast get hungry, but not severely. Drinking plain water or calorie-free flavored water should be more than enough to see you through 12 to 14 hours.

If you do get hungry, remember you're on a mission. You're not just cutting calories, you're specifically not having any calories for 12 hours, which is a terrific way of burning pounds, especially if you get up in the morning and have a healthy,

In regards to the mini-fast, and as with any general weight-loss advice, ask your doctor about its role for you, individually. People with diabetes, for example, may need to check their blood sugar more frequently during a mini-fast, or even adjust their medication. For people at risk of bulimia or other eating disorders, a mini-fast may not be advised. Again, check with your doctor for your own specific guidance.

protein-based breakfast. Your metabolism experiences a signifi-cant change, compared to that late-night snacking and either skipping breakfast or indulging in carbohydrates. Try it for a month. If the pounds aren't falling off, I'll have my friends at iMetabolic® send you a free box of protein bars. Seriously. (For iMetabolic® contact information, see Appendix F, Resources.)

49. Eat a protein bar

They're not just for athletes. Have a protein bar as a meal re-placement or in place of a snack you'd otherwise have eaten without thinking about it. Of course you're going to read the label first: The ideal protein bar will have about 150 to 200 cal-ories and 10 to 15 grams of protein. For a rundown on protein bars and their nutritional content, you can link to a blog post

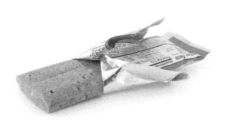

I've made on protein bars, at www. SasseGuide.com. So, how do you find the ideal bar? Experimentation. Try a few. Read the labels. Make sure you're not having a candy bar in disguise. Here's what to look for:

⬥ Natural ingredients. The fewer artificial ingredients, the better.

⬥ Vitamins and minerals. A nice source of what your body needs and a convenient way to get it.

⬥ Saturated fat should be less than 10 percent of total calo-ries (unless it comes from nuts.)

⬥ Protein. Bars need to have at least 10 grams.

⬥ Simple sugars. Less than 10 grams is best.

⬥ Calories should be between 100 and 250 for a snack. Above that, you're in meal replacement territory.

I've come to believe that protein bars are one of the greatest inventions ever. In the old days, most of them consisted of an astronomical amount of sugar and were probably flavored with high fructose corn syrup and dressed up with language on the packaging that hinted at healthy goodness, when in fact they were just a diabetes delivery vehicle.

Times have changed. New manufacturers have stepped into the void with tasty, good-for-you protein bars that start with a healthy dose of protein. From my point of view, the best of them keep the carbohydrates to a minimum and as a result have lower caloric contents, somewhere in the 150- to 230-calorie range. This seems just about right for most people as a breakfast or an afternoon snack when hunger is creeping in and willpower is charging out.

Protein bars with very low carbohydrates—less than 10 grams per bar—serve not only to provide an enjoyable, tasty snack but also suppress appetite for many hours.

50. Listen to your stomach

Who's hungry? Your stomach or your eyes? Eat only when your stomach is actually hungry and stop eating when your stomach is no longer empty. This is different than being full, which is a clue for three-year-olds to stop eating but not for intelligent adults trying to lose weight, maintain a healthy weight and live a better life. It may take 20 to 30 minutes for signals from the stomach to reach the brain and convince the brain the stomach is full. Stop eating when you're no longer actively hungry. Stop eating when you've had a small, reasonable portion and there is still food left on your plate. Then send the plate away as soon as you can reasonably (or politely) do so. Give the brain the time to get the message the stomach already knows: You've had enough.

51. Skip the dried fruit

Somewhere along the line everyone got the idea that dried fruit is an immensely healthy snack. But in the process of dehydrating and removing all the water from the fruit, what's produced is a very calorie-dense snack. A dried apricot has a great deal of concentrated sugar and calories per bite when compared to a fresh apricot.

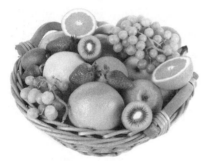

Instead of snacking on mummified fruit and getting a huge dose of calories with every bite, go for the fresh fruit, which has more bulk, more fiber, more water and fewer calories.

52. Eat frozen or freeze-dried fruit

Frozen fruits, on the other hand, are great alternatives to calming down that sweet tooth. Frozen fruit makes a great dessert or the answer to that sudden craving for something sweet. Bananas, berries, grapes, mangos, pineapples—simply wash and freeze and enjoy later. If you're buying commercially produced frozen fruit, read the label and make sure you're just getting the fruit, not fruit in sugary syrup.

Another alternative today is freeze-dried fruits and vegetables, which pack the original nutrient value of the fresh variety and offer a healthy dose of fiber while skipping the heavy calorie and carb components of dehydrated fruit.

53. Don't eat directly out of the box

It's like thinking outside the box, only different. Never eat food directly out of the container it comes in. Instead, pour a measured amount (try the exact serving size listed in the nutritional

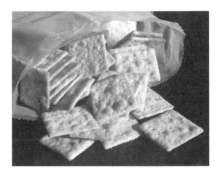

facts label, for an interesting and educational experience) onto a separate serving plate. Use a modest-sized plate or bowl, and close up the box or bag and return it to the pantry or refrigerator. Have a large glass of ice water with your snack and finish the snack with more water—not more snack.

54. Substitute the next processed snack with fresh fruit or vegetable

It's just as easy to peel an orange as it is to open a bag of chips, but it's a whole lot better for you. Or rinse some fresh carrots or raw broccoli or snow peas. You could substitute steamed vegetables, sure, but that requires rinsing, trimming, cutting, shaving, boiling the water and steaming the vegetables. If you have the time, definitely do this sometimes.

Fresh fruit and raw veggies require rinsing and eating. They're simple, satisfying and deliver natural vitamins. Granted, fresh fruit has a lot of sugar. You don't want to build your entire meal around it, because massive consumption of fruit would provide a huge carbohydrate intake, but some fresh fruit, not fruit juice, not fruit sugar snacks, not fruit-flavored ice cream, but fruit needs to be in your diet. It's good for you and it tastes great.

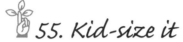

55. Kid-size it

If you absolutely cannot live without French fries (and you can, actually) then order kid-sized fries. If the food provider you're frequenting won't sell kid-sized to an adult, buy the small and throw some away. This works on any kind of indulgence, not just French fries. Never super-size anything. At the same time, avoid the items on the children's menu that seem set on promoting childhood obesity, such as those self-same French fries, or chicken fingers, juice boxes and desserts. But if you're indulging in something, kid-sized smaller portions or half portions fill the bill.

56. Eat in designated eating areas

Don't eat in front of the TV. Don't eat in your car. Don't eat while reading. Don't eat in front of the computer or while using the Internet. Eat only in designated eating areas such as the kitchen table or dining room. Yes, this takes the fun out of dinner and a movie happening simultaneously in your front room, but the upshot is you keep distractions to a minimum and can enjoy every bite you consume. In addition, you'll be aware of every bite you consume, and maybe you'll stop a little sooner.

And what's more, you'll stop all the unconscious calorie consumption taking place while your mind is focused on something else.

If you're watching a movie, enjoy the movie! If you must have something in your mouth, have some sugar-free gum or a glass of ice-water. You can eat later.

57. Make your own rules

Develop a personalized system of eating. Too many generic or one-size-fits-all diet plans fail to take into account the individual side of weight loss. No one knows your weaknesses better than you. If you simply have to have a candy bar once a day (and you don't, actually) write it into your rules for weight loss and work around it—find a way to balance those calories out by additional exercise or smaller meals at dinner.

I, for example, cannot live without chocolate. I know as a weight-loss doctor this is very weak of me, but I must admit that life would not be worth living for me without it. Does that mean I abandon healthy eating and give in to every temptation? No, I look forward to small treats of my absolute favorite chocolate, once in a while. I relish them. And then I go days or weeks without having any at all. I am quite sure that I enjoy chocolate ten times more now than I did when I was a kid and could eat as much as I wanted. And I make up for the treats with calorie cuts in other areas.

58. Be picky about what you eat

Don't waste your calories on a food or snack that is only so-so. Make sure you really enjoy the calories you're consuming. If you don't love the food you're eating, why eat it at all?

59. Pass the bread

Pass the bread. To someone else. Pass it to the end of the table. Distract yourself with conversation with your dinner companions while you're waiting for the waiter to take the orders and serve the food. The bread basket is one of the worst inventions of modern restaurants. By the time you get to dinner at a restaurant you're *hungry*. You've worked up an appetite and chanc-

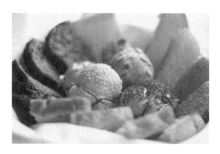

es are you haven't been somewhere like your own house (and pantry), where you could snack. The fact that you're already in a restaurant means portions will probably be larger than they need to be. And higher in calories and higher in carbs. Disaster.

The fact that you're hungry and facing a wait for dinner means temptations are larger than they need to be, too. And the wait staff has been trained to up-sell your meal, whether in the drive through ("Would you like fries with that?") or in the elegant four-star restaurant ("Can we suggest the five-cheese temptation on a plate?") Already your meal is threatening you with more calories than you need. Pass the bread basket to someone else. If everyone just keeps passing it you might even burn some calories.

60. Switch to Splenda or another sugar substitute

Take the sugar out of everything you can, and while you're doing so, take a look at Splenda, which is sugar, sort of, in a less harmful form.

Sugar is poison to an overweight person.

That sounds a little extreme, but look at the facts. Whether we're talking about sugar in the form of table sugar (sucrose) or high fructose corn syrup, sugar leads to a rapid surge in serum blood sugar and a subsequent rise in circulating hormones of insulin and leptin. More and more studies show that this cycle not only leads to resurgence of hunger in a very short time, but also triggers the metabolic processes that lead to obesity, diabetes, high blood pressure and metabolic syndrome (a disease comprised of a series of adverse conditions).

To a normal-weight person who isn't trying to lose weight, calling sugar "poison" sounds like hyperbole. To an overweight person who struggles daily with hunger and the fight against obesity, diabetes and other health problems associated with weight gain, sugar and all of the simple carbohydrates that metabolize immediately into blood sugar are, in fact, a type of poison. If you'd like more information on this topic, I have a blog post from August 21, 2008, on the metabolic syndrome (http://www.sasseguide.com/blog/sasse-guide-blog/) you can take a look at.

> "Diet and light brands are actually health and wellness brands."
>
> ~ Coca-Cola's chief executive, E. Neville Isdell (2007).

Sugar is a poison that acts in very slow motion. It tastes good, and it's unregulated. There's no skull and crossbones on the labels of products containing sugar. But if you've struggled with extra pounds and are engaged in the battle to lose weight, then it's important to take an aggressive stance toward sugar and simple carbs and their effects on your blood sugar. Avoid them. Work hard to avoid them. Count not only calories but carbs and keep that number low. Aim for less than 30 grams of sugar a day and understand that number adds up *fast*.

Sugar substitutes offer the chance to keep the taste of sugar in your foods—you can even cook with some of them—while cutting out some of the harmful effects. I'm aware that one day there may be proven adverse effects from these chemicals, too. But from a public health perspective, it strikes me as incredibly unlikely that any health problems uncovered in the future with these sugar substitutes will come close to rivaling the catastrophic health effects of obesity. A teaspoon of Splenda contains less than one gram of carbohydrate while a teaspoon of sugar contains four.

For more information on Splenda, check out http://www.gasdetection.com/news2/health_news_digest26.html

61. Switch to diet soda and zero-calorie beverages

Leaving your favorite soda behind is hard for the first week or two. But after that you'll probably find you'll never go back to sugared drinks.

Some of you may be asking about the chemicals in diet soda, and I share your concern—I'm not going to defend the chemical additives in food. But let's get some perspective. If you need to lose weight, sugar is a toxin for you. Sugar, excessive calories and, most definitely, calories from carbohydrates are the enemy.

So focus on the known enemy—sugar—as opposed to the potential enemy—sugar substitutes. If you're currently drinking beverages sweetened with sugar, it's time to stop. And reading almost any label from juice to soda, you'll find sodas, fruit juices, fruit punches and every other kind of non-diet soft drink contains an enormous amount of refined sugar in the form of sucrose or high fructose corn syrup. Eliminate these drinks from your diet, by whatever means necessary.

And if the idea of imbibing those chemicals really bothers you, switch to water. No one says you have to have sugar *or* sugar substitutes.

That three-soda-a-day habit may seem hard to give up, but it's substantially easier than almost any other changes you will make.

A very good friend of mine, a physician I've worked with for many years, made the switch to diet sodas. He'd been drinking four full-sugar Cokes a day and laughed at me when I suggested his goal of losing 30 pounds would be best achieved by eliminating those drinks immediately. Over the course of the next several months, he gradually came to accept my advice and one day he told me he was making the switch. He was skeptical and thought it would take years to get over sugared sodas, but in fact, within 10 days he had no desire to go back from diet. Whether this is a testament to the great power of modern chemistry to create sweeteners that taste good or to an individual's commitment to dropping sugar from his diet, it doesn't matter. The net result is my friend did lose the 30 pounds over the next four months, almost entirely as a result of that one change made to his diet.

62. Get the Skinny on the Carbs You're Consuming

Not all carbs are created equal. Some are far worse than others, meaning they have a simple molecular formula, cause larger spikes in blood sugars and insulin and are absorbed faster, leading to more weight gain. The Glycemic Index is an database you can access that ranks foods on a scale from 0 to 100. Low GI foods are those that spike blood sugars the least, causing the least weight gain. The higher the GI number, the worse choice the food is if you're trying to lose weight. Low-glycemic index diets have been shown to improve both glucose and lipid (circulating fat in the bloodstream) levels in people with both diabetes type 1 and type 2, and can reduce insulin levels and insulin resistance, as well as helping to reduce appetite and delay hunger because of their slow digestion and absorption. If you want to get an idea of what you're eating before you eat it, check out the database at www.glycemicindex.com.

63. Limit alcohol intake

Studies have shown that in moderation, one drink a day is beneficial to your health. A small glass of red wine is probably

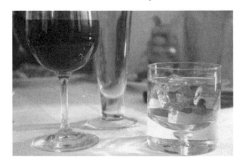

the ticket, because red wine contains the newly identified healthy substance called Resveritrol. Any single alcoholic drink per day is probably beneficial based on new actuarial data, but wine seems to be the best and drinking one 3- to 4-ounce glass a day can reduce the health risk of insulin and glucose-related diseases such as diabetes. But the calories in alcohol are unhealthy, especially in excess, and especially when drinking to excess makes you more prone to overindulging mindlessly, adding more and more health ramifications.

64. Have a cup of tea

Tea is a great drink, nutritious and full of health benefits, especially green tea. Studies have shown that green tea may prevent or improve obesity and possibly reduce the risk of associated diseases, including diabetes and coronary heart disease.

Green tea may not be the proven wonder-drink its proponents might like us to believe, but there is at least enough theoretical backing to support its health benefits to give it a try. That doesn't mean that you can add sugar or cream or other calories to your tea or drink it in large amounts; and this isn't a permission slip for calorie-rich, if delicious, drinks like Thai iced tea (a high-calorie, sweet, dessert-like milky and delicious tea). But go ahead and have a cup of tea, enjoy the relaxation, take the time to decompress and reduce stress. But use only zero-calorie sweeteners.

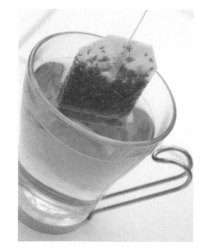

And interestingly, caffeinated teas may not be too bad to drink either. Caffeine acts as a mild stimulant and mild appetite suppressant. For a person seeking to lose weight, increase activity and improve health, some caffeine is clearly beneficial. No one knows for certain how much caffeine is the ideal amount, but certainly 100 to 200mg per day is exceedingly unlikely to be harmful and may help.

The Multiplier Effect

Imagine you substitute Carrots (30 kcal) for your usual snack of a Snickers Bar (273 kcal) every workday afternoon. Over the course of the year you cut out 60,750 kcal and just lost 17 pounds!

Human beings, by changing the inner attitudes of their minds,
can change the outer aspects of their lives.

—William James

Become a possibilitarian. No matter how dark things seem to be or actually are, raise your sights and see possibilities —always see them, for they're always there.

—Norman Vincent Peale

The Working Life

Most of us spend about a third of our days at work, which can be hazardous to our health, or at least to our waistlines. There doesn't seem to be any profession that's immune to the allure of food at work. Dentist's offices and banks give away suckers. Offices celebrate events and occasions with cake and pot lucks. Even construction workers, who should be safe out in the field, are offered food by rolling caterers often charmingly called "roach coaches" (there's a tempting name—how can anyone resist?)

Short of winning the lottery and never going to work again, you'll need to have some defenses against the siren call of work food.

65. Move the candy bowl

Out of sight is out of mind. Studies have shown if the candy bowl is at least six feet away from a person, that person dips into it less often and eats less. This isn't a tough concept—when the candy bowl is within easy reach, there's no thought involved in reaching over and having something sweet. It's mindless eating, and just seeing the bowl can stimulate temptation. If you're there all day with that candy bowl staring at you, temptation is going to be pretty hard to resist.

Now think about moving the candy bowl. You're going to have to get up out of your chair to get to it. You'll have to make an affirmative decision to have a piece of candy. And whether it's true or not, you're going to imagine everyone around you is aware you're getting another piece of candy. Nothing wrong with a little bit of negative peer pressure at this point. Make it harder on yourself—put the candy bowl at least six feet away. Out of your line of sight. Not on a convenient route between you and the washroom or you and your other duties. And fill it with candy that requires a whole process of unwrapping to eat it. You'll find in no time your consumption of mindlessly eaten candy has been reduced significantly.

Obstacles are those frightening things that become visible when we take our eyes off our goals."

—Henry Ford

66. Get rid of the candy bowl

What's stopping you? Unless there's some kind of weird mandate in your office that there must be a candy bowl, you might find you're doing everyone a favor, from the mailman who always dips in, to the customers who find themselves waiting in the office, to your coworkers who might be relieved when the temptation is removed. And you'll be removing your own temptation to graze the entire time you're working.

Removing the candy bowl is a simple move that can result in a substantial reduction of needless carbohydrate calories over the course of the year. It's a simple move, but it can empower you to make other, similar moves.

Think about places in your life where you're faced with other, metaphorical candy bowls—the pastry platter at your office (or the open box of doughnuts), the constantly replenished snacks in your pantry or the bag of treats you keep in your car "just in case." Whatever the source of constant temptation in your life, work to eliminate it. Once it's gone you'll realize how constant and harmful the constant temptation was.

67. Pack some sugar-free gum

Many people work in an environment that involves lots of lunch meetings, dinner meetings or travel. This is one of the toughest challenges for avoiding temptation and high-calorie, high-carbohydrate foods and goodies.

One of the most common workplace problems I see is when a person must attend a lunch meeting or, worse, attend dinner meetings several times a week. Food is often served buffet-style, almost always rich in calories and carbs. Lunch buffets rarely fail to provide the ever-tempting dessert, and who can resist the piece of chocolate cake at the end of a boring lunch meeting? You did your penance, right? Stayed awake through the whole meeting, didn't you? Then go on, you deserve a little treat.

No. Plain and simple, this is a formula for disaster and steady weight gain. You need a battle plan that lets you get through the meetings without succumbing to temptations put in front of you several times a week.

For starters, bring some sugar-free gum to every meeting. Use it like a weapon against hunger and temptation. Grab your small portion of healthy choices, sit down, eat up, and then pop the sugar-free gum in your mouth before any more food can find its way onto your plate or into your mouth. You'll coast through the meeting and be out of there before dessert catches you.

68. Do the talking

When you attend meetings, it is time for you to do the talking. Ask more questions, give a presentation, get involved. Career move? Maybe. But this is a weight-loss book: The more you're talking and engaged, the less you're eating.

While others are heading back to the trough for seconds and the dessert plate, you walk up and engage the keynote speaker. Ask the company VP about your department's goals, shake hands with a colleague. Interact with the humans present and not with the food. You may find you not only lose the pounds but improve your standing at work.

69. Fight the working blues

Construction workers, mechanics and other people involved in physical jobs can find the job site a tough place to maintain a focus on healthy eating habits. Not only do temptations from doughnuts in the job trailer to a couple beers after work abound, but food choices are often unhealthy because there's such a restricted time for lunch. Given 30 minutes to go forage, find and eat, a lot of people are going to head straight for fast food or a sandwich shop or even the deli in a grocery store. It's fast, cheap and easy. To make it worse, you've probably worked up a big appetite and want to indulge it before taking on the afternoon's work.

If you can work hard at your job, you can work hard at the fight against obesity as well. Take five minutes in the morning or the night before and you can bring a sack lunch and know all the carbs and calories you're about to eat. A chicken sandwich beats a burger in the weight-loss arena. Even better, the rotisserie chicken from the grocery store can provide several days-worth of lunches. Bring fresh veggies or fruit or a pre-made salad. Bring a thermos of water rather than picking up a mountain-sized soft drink at the convenience store. And if you get to the end of lunch and still feel hungry, give it 20 minutes and see if you don't feel sated. It takes that long for the message "satisfied" to reach the brain, and you might find starting up again after lunch easier without the grease, salt and fat from the burger slowing you down.

Weight loss is an ongoing battle. If you've been eating lunch with the crew, explain what you're doing— they just might join you, especially when it starts working and you start losing weight.

Keep away from people who try to belittle your ambitions.
Small people always do that, but the really great make you feel
that you, too, can become great.

—Mark Twain

The Working-Out Life

At the end of the day, at the end of the year and at the end of your next decade, it will be an incontrovertible truth that *calories in* roughly equals *calories out*. I say roughly because there are always some individual differences in the way calories are processed and metabolized, but those are small compared to the overall grand equation that tells us *energy in* equals *energy out*. So cut the calories going in and increase the energy going out, whenever you can, however you can.

You receive an immense benefit from increasing the energy or calories your body burns through increased activity and exercise. And while there are many ways to talk ourselves out of a big, involved workout regimen, there are no good reasons we can't start small and start today. Walking and using light, hand-held dumbbells are enormously effective, and easy, ways to start increasing muscle use and healthy calorie burn.

Once you start exercising, you'll feel better, you'll feel more energetic, and you'll want to do more of it. So start. Just start. No matter how small the effort, just begin and good things will begin to happen.

70. Just get there

OK, so you don't always feel like working out. Make a deal with yourself. Just put on your shoes and sit on the exercise bike or stand on the treadmill or elliptical. What happens next is up to you.

For most of us, of course, what happens next is that we do a little exercise, take a few turns on the bicycle or a few steps on the step machine. And a few steps leads to a few more steps. I have on occasion managed to get a whole workout in on a day when I could not imagine finding the time nor the willpower, just by making a deal that lacing up my shoes and getting to the machine was all I really had to do.

71. Up the ante

Once you're on the exercise equipment, make a deal with yourself to stay there as long as your workout would have been. No one says you have to work out. Just stay there. After a while, working out will be better than standing or sitting immobile.

The Multiplier Effect

Let's say you started taking a 20 minute walk at lunch every day at work. At a moderate pace of 3mph, that burns around 73 kcal. Over the year, guess what? You just lost another 5 pounds.

---

72. Make exercise fun

Do whatever it takes to get yourself into the habit of exercising. Work out with a friend or loved one. Try new things. Go rollerblading. Try golfing. Go dancing. Make your workout time a time you can spend with someone you enjoy spending time with.

If you're going it alone, find something you love. Love to shop? How many times can you power-walk through the mall? Or if you love to read, try finding books on CD and transferring them onto your iPod or even using a disc player. Always loved swashbuckling movies? Try fencing for your workout. There's more to working out than running or walking or bench press. Find what you enjoy and you'll have a much better chance of sticking with it.

73. Build your exercise program gradually

By developing an actual program and knowing what to expect out of yourself, you will find a greater degree of comfort and a better chance of avoiding injury. If you can keep your initial efforts at a reasonable level of intensity—that is to say, don't jump in with both feet with whatever you choose to do—you have a better chance of succeeding as your workout grows longer and you spend more time exercising.

Increase your amount of activity weekly, by no more than 10 percent. For instance, start by walking 10 minutes a day and move up gradually to 30 sustainable minutes. If you're walking, you might want to pick up five minutes every couple days.

74. Have an alternate plan

If your choice of exercise takes you outdoors, have a backup plan for inclement weather. If your workout buddy is going to

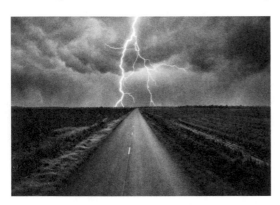

be gone for a while, invite another friend to join you for a week. Or keep track of everything you do to impress your friend when you're working out together again. Don't let "circumstances beyond your control" take control of your workouts.

75. Avoid rebound weight gain: work out with weights

We've already said that one of the keys to weight loss is to use and build your muscle. Studies show that people who diet tend to burn storage of both fat *and* muscle. This is a problem when the diet ends and the dieter experiences intense hunger that, if satisfied, leads to rebound weight gain. To avoid rebound weight gain you need to build and preserve lean body mass (your muscle mass). The only way to do that is to use those muscles, strengthening them by lifting as many times a week as you can (at least three or four).

Buy a pair of five-pound hand weights and use them whenever you're idle, like when you're watching television or on the phone. Even a beginner can get a high number of repetitions of each movement with such a light weight and without being overly sore the next day. Before long you're probably going to find yourself wanting to try something other than curls (maybe something for the triceps or the shoulders or back or chest) and you're going to start thinking about graduating to 10-pound weights. If you've never picked up a pair of weights and you don't have a trainer handy to show you proper form, you can pick up information on lifting at http://exercise.about.com/cs/exbeginners/a/begstrength.htm and take a look at Appendix D for some workout suggestions from iMetabolic®.

The point isn't to turn you into an Olympic athlete or a bodybuilder. The point is to make you a weight lifter in the sense of being someone who does resistance training on a regular basis. Three to five days a week of 50 to 100 repetitions with a set of very light hand weights will do wonders.

Anaerobic exercise (weight lifting) stimulates the body chemistry to support, maintain and grow lean body mass. It creates muscle, which burns calories more efficiently than fat, requiring the metabolism to kick in and burn fat stores to preserve and promote the protein building blocks. This type of exercise signals, biochemically, that 'this is an active person' and an active person needs protein and muscle to be maintained 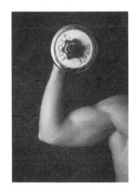 This type of active body needs fat stores to be burned. It does not need giant levels of insulin and leptin and giant stores of fat tucked away in every corner, crevice, roll and fold. Use your muscles daily. Your body will love you for it. *You* will love you for it. (For more in-depth information on weight-bearing exercise, lean body mass and avoiding rebound weight-gain, take a look at the article on Rebound Weight Gain Blamed for Diets Failing in Appendix F.)

76. When you watch TV, keep moving

Studies have shown individuals only burn about 68 calories an hour while sitting (Levine, 2005) whereas they burn more than twice as many by standing and pacing.

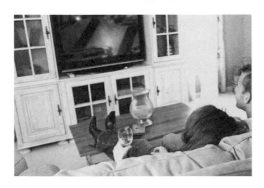

We all watch TV. I work more than 100 hours a week seeing patients, advising, performing surgery, writing and speaking, and somehow I still find time to watch TV. The problem is it's too easy to get lost in what you're watching so that a couple hours can go by and you haven't moved (except maybe to get something to eat). The TV is entertaining, the couch is comfortable, the combination is sublime.

Break the sedentary pattern. Instead of getting comfortable, curling up on the couch and firing up the high def TV, try *doing something*. Just imagine if during the entire two hours you were watching TV you were also exercising, even if only mildly. The result would be a substantial caloric burn. Now multiply that caloric burn out times an entire week of TV watching and then times an entire year of TV watching. Think you don't have time to work out? You've just snuck in somewhere from seven to 14 hours in a single week and not even noticed because you were entranced by what you were watching. Making the change to walking, pacing or just keeping active during your TV time, you will lose more than 10 pounds in a year.

It's your life. Make a bold choice. Take out the couch altogether and replace it with a piece of exercise equipment. Or move the TV to wherever the stationary bike, treadmill, elliptical machine or stair-climber is in your house. Eliminate the comfortable seats and vary your routine, doing different exercises every day—something other than sitting and resting. The same goes for any sedentary activity—if you're spending time on the phone, get up and pace. Move around. Phones are cordless now; you're free to move about. Do so.

77. Burn more calories than you eat

Most people who want to lose weight eat too much and move too little. When it comes to weight loss, it might be easier to think of your mission in terms of finding simple ways to burn more calories every day. Try this: Get up 15 minutes earlier than you have to and watch 15 minutes less of television every night and you've created 30 minutes during the day when you can exercise and burn more calories and lose more weight.

The more ways, large and small, that you can burn calories during your day, the more weight you will lose over the course of the year. Let the multiplier effect work in your favor for a change.

One of the most challenging parts of losing weight and keeping it off involves the meals we eat at restaurants and on the road. The food is richer and tastier, the alcohol is flowing, the portions are larger and with business colleagues or friends and family, the desire to kick back, relax and enjoy the surroundings, the company—and the food.

It takes a solid battle plan, but you can lose weight and keep it off even if you eat out regularly. It takes commitment and discipline, just like everything important in life, but the results are worth it.

78. Limit restaurant meals

Americans eat out four to five times a week. Even without the temptations found in restaurants, Americans consume 3,790 calories a day according to USA Year Book 2000-2002 (http://www.diet-blog.com/archives/2006/12/27/do_americans_eat_3790_calories_per_day.php). And, yes, everyone is busy and it's easier to catch a bite to eat in the nearest fast food restaurant for lunch and takeout for dinner. It is easy. It's also unhealthy.

Fortunately, there are healthy alternatives.

◇ You can find countless healthy recipes in cookbooks and on cooking Web sites that take 30 minutes or less to prepare.

◇ You can precook a week's worth of meals, including lunches you can take to the office and dinners you can warm up in no time. I usually make Sunday my cooking day and involve the whole family. We'll make batches of soup and freeze them, and I often bring soup to the office for lunch.

◇ If you (or your family) aren't culinary-minded (or if the results would be off-putting), there are personal chef services that will do everything from meeting with you to setting up a menu, shopping for ingredients and preparing a week's worth of food at a time. The service might be pricey but your health is worth it—and you'll be saving money by not eating out all week.

◇ Crockpot cooking is a great alternative to eating out. Dump water or broth, vegetables and lean meats into the crockpot in the morning, and dinner's ready when you get home in the evening. For healthy crockpot recipes, check out www.chefdave.org.

79. Traveling on the road: Bring your good intentions with you

If one of your downfalls is lots of dinners out on the road, it's time to change your philosophy.

You travel for business, lug your bags around and work hard to earn a living. You deserve some dinners out with nice food and dessert, right? Wrong! Calories on the road count just as much as calories at home. More so if businesses lunches and dinners take you into restaurants more often than at home. So travel smart: Pack your weight-loss intentions, your goals, your willpower and your workout clothes. Wear your running shoes to meetings and schedule your meetings around your walk, run or weight-lifting regimen. Most hotels have gym facilities and most restaurants have healthy choices.

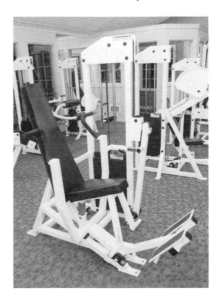

🌱 80. Eat _before_ eating out

That sounds like a bad idea, doesn't it? But how often have you gone out for dinner only to discover there's a delay before you're seated or even that your last meal was longer ago than you thought and even though you're seated as soon as you arrive, you're starving. And _everything_ on the menu looks good. This is not a good time to be confronted with a menu full of unhealthy opportunities.

Eat _before_ you dine out. Just take the edge off the hunger so you can make reasonable and responsible meal choices. Have a protein bar or shake, a piece of fruit or a vegetable snack. Then face the menu with courage. And determination. Because this tip only works if you can truly exercise discipline and not barrel ahead with a full five-course dinner anyway. The best defense is a good offense.

🌱 81. Drink water

Water, water, water. Drinking water before you eat will help fill you up. Drink plenty of it. Many weight-loss plans fail due to the lack of hydration. Without plenty of water, you're thirstier and probably hungrier. Although water probably does very little to trigger the body's chemical or hormonal signals of fullness, drinking plenty of water undoubtedly helps you feel fuller faster and gives you something besides high-calorie food to put in your mouth.

82. Reduce portion sizes

Restaurant plates and the portions on top of them have increased 20 percent in size over the past decade and the calories in restaurant meals have increased much more than that, in most cases. Fast food meals are being super-sized. In many restaurants, bigger is considered better. When you're eating at home you have choices. You can choose smaller plates, weigh and measure food choices and read labels carefully to determine serving sizes.

When you're eating in a restaurant, remember you're the guest and the restaurant and its staff the merchant. They're working for you. Ask for what you want, whether that's smaller portions, less sauce or substituting unhealthy side dishes for healthier choices (or even withholding them altogether).

83. Avoid sitting near food

Have you ever started eating again after a satisfying meal even though you're not really hungry? It's just because the food is sitting right there in front of you. How much worse can this be if you're at a buffet where the food never goes away? So if you find yourself at a buffet, sit across the room from it. If serving dishes are left on the table in a restaurant or at a friend's house, move them arm's length away from you.

Once the meal is finished, relocate to a new place, to a new activity, to something that does not involve food. If you're visiting with friends and conversing, then make the after-dinner activity a nice long walk. Don't sit around on the comfortable chairs and dip back into the appetizers and leftovers.

Only he who can see the invisible can do the impossible.

—Frank L. Gaines

84. Never super-size, even if it's cheaper

Some restaurants offer specials, such as extra-large for the price of a large or two-for-one. Super-sizing your meal just means adding meaningless calories to your diet, calories you weren't planning on eating and won't miss if you never have.

85. Don't order extras

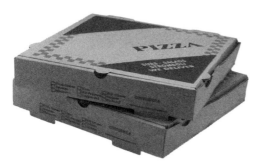

"Would you like fries with that?" No, probably not. And just because your food comes with a choice of bread and two side orders and a free soda doesn't mean you have to take it. Just order the meal you were planning on eating in the first place. Or less.

86. Just say no to refills

"Can I get you another one of those?" Don't get sucked into accepting free refills of anything with calories, food or drink. At restaurants, try asking for water after you finish the first soda. If it's soda, make sure it's zero-calorie every time.

Avoid two-for-one take-out restaurant deals. It's hard to pass up a bargain—look at what a great deal this is!—but your body has to store all those extra calories as fat, and fat takes a toll on your health, probably more quickly than you expect. So that good deal isn't such a good deal after all.

87. Bring your own to-go box and plan to use it

If you can't stand seeing food go to waste, bring your own to-go box (any food-storage container will do and is a more eco-friendly option than the to-go box the restaurant will provide.) Plan on using it because you're planning not to eat everything on your plate. Just because you paid for a meal doesn't mean you have to eat all of it. In fact, the best bargain out there is paying for one meal, but getting to eat two, with leftovers for lunch the next day.

88. Organize a supper club instead of going out to eat

Get together with friends who like to cook healthy meals and are passionate about maintaining their own healthy weight (or are even in the weight-loss process like you are.) Exchange healthy recipes, eat wonderful food and enjoy good companionship. At the end of the meal, you don't even have to tip (though you might want to offer to help clean up.)

89. Plan ahead for being a dinner guest

Ask the host or hostess what will be served. For one thing, it can help you decide what wine or zero-calorie beverage to bring as a gift. For another, you can plan ahead of time what extra workouts you might need to burn the night's calories or how to avoid certain foods you know you don't want to eat.

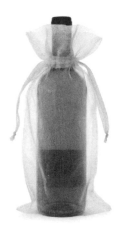

According to etiquette experts, as a dinner guest it's impolite to be a picky eater or overly concerned with the calorie content of what you're being served. But if you're seriously trying to lose weight, and if you're social and eat meals with friends frequently, following the rules of etiquette could derail all your hard work.

Don't feel compelled to eat everything in order to be a good guest. Eat lightly, praise lavishly and leave something on your plate. Skip dessert and pass on the bread and tell them you wish you had room for more but you're really quite stuffed.

90. Avoid temptation when "family" means "food"

Being a guest can be difficult. Being a guest on a diet can be even more difficult. But being a guest for family functions is sometimes the hardest test of all. Everyone in the family thinks they know you, what you like to eat and how much. When you start making changes it will confuse and possibly alarm them. They'll want the old you back. They'll want to feed the old you.

Whether your family meets once a year for a major holiday or every Sunday for a traditional family dinner, you need to take control of what you're going to eat. Try to mentally prepare before going. Know ahead of time if you're going to be facing dietary choices, like potatoes for vegetables or breaded meats for the main course, and look for ways to lessen the caloric hit, from taking smaller portions to planning the workouts to make up for it. You might want to try a mini-fast that night, or curtail your calories for the next couple days.

In addition, if you've made dessert a special occasion rather than a nightly expectation, this is no time to change. Even if you've anticipated your father's breaded shrimp or your

mother-in-law's potatoes au gratin, you don't have to eat the unexpected seven-layer German chocolate cake. Skipping dessert isn't that unusual anymore. You might even have other family members joining you.

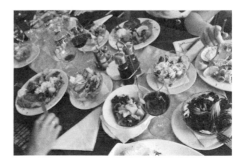

You've got to say, I think that if I keep working at this and want it badly enough I can have it. It's called perseverance.

—Lee Iacocca

Food for Thought

Some of the most important changes you'll make on your weight-loss journey will happen within your own mind, invisible to others. These changes begin with a new appreciation of the importance of you: your health, your body, your life and your goals.

91. Visualize the New you

Pretend you've already accomplished your weight-loss goals. Close your eyes and visualize. Stop and let the feeling pervade your senses. What do you feel? Proud, more fit, healthier, strong. Now remind yourself of that feeling every morning. Take time and really let it sink in. We are what we think.

92. Be your own boss

Be the "boss" of what goes into your mouth. Blaming others for your own overeating is a way of avoiding personal responsibility. In the end, no one can lose your weight for you. As long as no one is holding your nose and force-feeding you, the choice is up to you. Just because your best friend or favorite relative baked something special doesn't mean you have to eat it. Take charge of your own life and take control of your own weight-loss.

93. Learn to turn celebration food away—gracefully

People love to cook for people they love. Holidays, birthdays and special occasions for some people means baking, and it's hard to say no to such honestly, lovingly prepared treats.

Learn to refuse food effectively and gracefully, even when pressured by others. Just say no to "Just try a bite" whether it's a special treat concocted to celebrate your accomplishments or birthday cake for someone in the office.

Make a statement to yourself and throw out that example of someone else's culinary good intentions. Thank them, tell them you'll enjoy it later and dispose of it. Down the disposal or into the trash with the coffee grounds and tuna cans. You can do it. Taking charge and being in control will feel better than giving in to temptation.

If you can imagine it, you can achieve it;
if you can dream it, you can become it.

—William Arthur Ward

94. Customize

Choose the eating plan, exercise plan and behavioral plan that you can live with. Initially you and your physician will construct an aggressive weight-loss plan. But it's the plan that you can live with, the plan that takes your individual lifestyle into account, that will keep the weight off long-term.

You must know yourself, and in time you'll learn what you can live with and what you can't. Try not to commit to an overly aggressive plan you know you can't live with. No point in setting yourself up for cheating and disappointment. On the other hand, find creative ways to embrace the program with some acknowledged exceptions. For example if the plan calls for absolutely no desserts all month, perhaps you agree to one 3-oz piece of dark chocolate per week as a reward for complying.

95. Learn new ways to eat

Reduce stress and then eat. Don't use eating as a stress-release device. Take a five-minute walk or stair-climb before lunch. Take a shower or read a book before dinner. Whatever you do to de-stress, do it before you eat so that eating itself isn't the stress reducer. It's a simple formula: Stress reduction = weight reduction.

96. Change the channel

The average American kid sees between 30 and 50 hours of food commercials on television every year, 90 percent of them advertising junk food. Children watch an average of 1,680 minutes of television a week—that's 28 hours they're not burning a whole lot of calories, but they are getting a whole lot of messages about what's tasty but not necessarily healthy. If the average American child is seeing that much television, the average American adult can't be far behind—or maybe even ahead. That's a lot of information you're absorbing about foods that aren't weight-loss healthy!

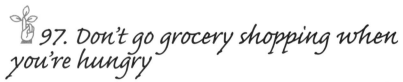

If you have to watch TV (and you don't) the next time some temptation appears on the screen that you and those you love would be better off without, *change the channel*. You don't have to let these purveyors of portliness into your home to parade their images of fat and carbs and calories. Just change the channel. You can always change back in 30 seconds.

97. Don't go grocery shopping when you're hungry

Everything looks more appetizing when you're hungry! Even broccoli and especially those quick-to-satisfy simple carbohydrates in shiny packages. Plus, when you're already hungry your willpower is at its lowest ebb. Why set yourself up for failure?

Plan for your grocery shopping trips. Figure out what you're having for dinner for the next week or so and figure out what ingredients you need for those meals. Your fruits and vegetables will be fresher, as well as your dairy products, if you're shopping more often and closer to when you use the products.

Eating something healthy will take the edge off hunger so you're not so tempted by all the treats on display. And if you absolutely have to run to the store at the last minute for a missing ingredient in tonight's healthy meal, make sure you're really running—in and out with no time to pick up something you don't need. Your body will thank you for it.

98. Learn when to shop

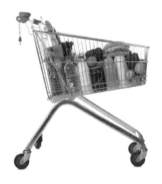

If you don't buy it, you can't eat it. Shop when stores are not crowded and you're not tempted to throw any old thing into the cart just so you can get out of there. Alternately, shopping when stores aren't crowded means you're not going to be distracted by all the noise and confusion—so no excuse for accidentally slipping in a packet of cookies or a tub of ice cream.

99. Make a list

Before you go to the grocery store, when you've determined what you're having for dinner in the next week and what safe, sane, healthy breakfast foods you need, write it all down and don't deviate from the list. Stay out of the junk food aisles, avoiding the crackers, cookies, chips, ice cream and packaged foods areas. The only appropriate spontaneous additions to the list should be the healthy things you forgot to write down or extra tempting fruits or vegetables.

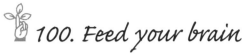 100. Feed your brain

Try listening to some motivational messages and information on weight loss during your commute. Try www.audiodiets.com for scientifically based weight-loss tools, information and motivation. This is your chance to control what goes into your brain and into your consciousness. Counteract the high fructose corn syrup, high-fat snack messages coming from the television by listening to messages that will help you achieve your goals. If the messages contained in advertising work—and they must work, or why would advertisers spend all that money to create those messages—then why not make listening to messages work for you? Control what you listen to and go for the good stuff.

101. Get a massage

Massage is an ancient, relaxing, therapeutic treatment that increases the brain's awareness of the body. I find many of my patients have lost touch with their own bodies, their own uniqueness and experiences. A massage enlivens dormant muscles and reminds them of the power and physicality of their own bodies and lives.

A massage can remind you of the connections between what you do in life, what you eat how your body reaches the shape it's in, how you experience appearance and sensation. I recommend as your journey commences and you begin to pay more attention to your body, your health and your nutrition, that you get a massage at least once a month. Yes, it feels indulgent. It feels great. Make it your reward for a job well done on your weight-loss program. And you've got permission—this is a doctor's recommendation.

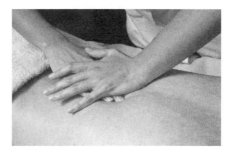

I learned that courage was not the absence of fear,
but the triumph over it. The brave man is not he who
does not feel afraid, but he who conquers that fear.

—Nelson Mandela

The only lifelong, reliable motivations are those that come from within, and one of the strongest of those is the joy and pride that grow from knowing that you've just done something as well as you can do it.

—Lloyd Dobens

Bonus Tips

1. Take it one day at a time

Don't be disheartened or overwhelmed by the enormity of your goals. Set realistic goals and wake each day looking forward to a successful day of maintaining your weight-management efforts. You didn't gain the weight overnight, and you won't lose it overnight, but you can lose it steadily by not looking too far ahead. Worry about tomorrow when it gets here. Today only concentrate on eating better and feeling better today. You've already set your goals—they'll lead you where you want to go step by step. Don't be overwhelmed by trying to accomplish everything at once.

2. Exercise your self-control

Learn to put your health and body weight desires above your food intake desires. Remind yourself of your goals and your mission and when you successfully navigate your way past a trap, congratulate yourself. Say "Good job!" and add your name to the statement and bask in the moment. That glow of accomplishment will help you avoid the next temptation even better. Plus, if you know temptation lurks in the form of a favorite taco stand or the food court at the mall or the corner candy store, reroute your route and avoid it! Out of sight is out of mind.

3. Eat mindfully

Be aware of what you're about to eat and when and why. Are you eating between meals because you're hungry or because you're bored? Are you putting food in your mouth just because you see it when you pass through a certain room in your house or office? Remove the temptation or reroute the way you move through spaces. Eat because you intended to eat, not because you were doing something else and fell into eating unconsciously.

The difference between the impossible and the possible lies in a person's determination.

—Tommy Lasorda

4. Figure out how much it costs you to remain overweight

Before you wonder if you can spend money on weight-loss programs or on a medically approved nutrition program, sit down and do the math and figure out what you're already spending by being overweight.

Yes, there are costs to carrying around excess weight. Add up what it costs to eat every week, including every meal, every coffee, every dessert, every snack, every meal at a restaurant, every trip to a convenience store. Then add in the cost of medications to treat problems caused by weight gain: headaches, backaches, heartburn, not to mention more serious (and expensive) problems such as diabetes and high blood pressure. Think about job opportunities you may have missed because an employer was looking for candidates with healthier weights in order to cut down on the costs of insurance. Not to mention once you have the job, studies have shown skinnier, healthy-weight or normal-weight people are paid more, on average, and have more chances for promotions and better jobs.

Think past the money. There are non-financial costs associated with being overweight, including costs of time, health and quality of life. You are too important to lose time, either to poor health or an early death. You don't deserve to suffer bad health and experience a lower quality of life when you could be feeling more fit, stronger, healthier and happier. So spend some time here. Figure out the costs. And then invest in *you*. You deserve it.

5. Make use of amazing healthy recipes

There is nothing more disheartening than trying to force yourself to stick to a diet that tastes lousy. Let's face it; no one is going to enjoy life if we take away all the good stuff to eat. Fortunately Chef Dave Fouts and Vicki Bovee, RD have thought of that and have put together many sample recipes to get your started. Some of my favorites are included in Appendix A of this book. Enjoy!

6. Jump start your weight loss with meal replacement shakes

I know, a liquid diet does not sound all that appealing, but wait until you see the pounds come off! Then your attitude will change quickly, and you'll say those shakes don't taste too bad after all.

The truth is that most medically-based weight-loss programs for those looking to lose significant weight utilize some version of a liquid meal replacement program for a period of weeks or months to quickly and efficiently peel off the pounds in a healthy way. This "Induction" weight-loss program is highly effective, accomplishing rapid weight loss in a healthy way while preserving the protein and nutrients your body needs. Nearly everyone who does this finds that the appetite suppression of the shakes works to block hunger and allow most people to stick with it for many weeks, or even months, without complaining. (Okay, maybe a few complaints, but the weight loss is worth it.)

Meal replacement shakes are protein-based, and provide a blend of nutrients including vitamins and minerals, and a modest amount of fat and carbs, to suppress appetite and allow the body to drop pounds in a healthy way. By eliminating the choices of "real foods" for a period of time, say six to twelve weeks, the meal replacement shakes serve as a very effective jump start to your successful weight-loss journey.

Appendix B, describes a safe and effective 1000 calorie per day diet that combines meal replacement shakes with some healthy fruits and a few real foods. An even stricter 800 calorie "shakes-only" plan can be very effective in a medically-supervised setting.

7. Imagine

How often do you suppose a sharpshooter would hit the target without taking the time to aim? What if the shooter fired randomly without clearly visualizing the target and thinking about the distance, speed, trajectory and factors involved in making the shot? Would the shooter hit the target at all?

Ask yourself: What is your target? Losing weight? Being healthier?

Now take aim.

One of the most important goals in your life is to lose the excess weight and maintain a healthy weight as you become a healthier person with a positive outlook, someone who looks better, feels better and lives longer. To achieve that goal and hit that target, you need to visualize clearly what you're trying to achieve and picture it clearly in your mind.

Take time every day to imagine what you will look and feel like once you've achieved your goal and hit your target. Force your mind to focus on feelings and actions associated with healthy living, healthy eating, a trimmer waistline and a better quality of life.

As we continue to concentrate on our goals and how to achieve them, we slowly and cumulatively continue to act, behave and think in ways both large and small that move us closer to achieving those goals. In short, we become what we imagine we can become.

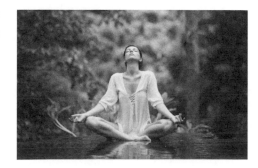

Conclusion

Losing weight and keeping it off is never easy. But there are ways to make it easier, things you can do to assure your success on this path you have chosen. You've just read 106 number of tips, every which of which is an action you can take.

We are all surrounded by messages that encourage us to eat more, entertain ourselves more and exercise less. We are surrounded by temptations to enjoy unhealthy treats and sumptuous high-calorie meals. And many of us are surrounded by people who are only too happy to encourage us to eat more, have a second helping, abandon that diet plan, have another handful of chips, watch the game, have another beer.

We have to fight back. Today the world is full of unprecedented amounts of food. Calories are everywhere and most of them taste good. Unless you are actively fighting to reduce your calorie and carbohydrate intake, you will keep gaining weight.

Make the multiplier effect work in your favor for a change. Make some small alterations in your daily routine that cut the calories you take in, and increase the calories you burn with exercise.

Then see those 10-calorie, 100-calorie or 300-calorie changes magnified when multiplied out over a year. Imagine you consumed 150 calories less each day by throwing out the top bun of every burger, passing on the bread bowl and eating fewer starches. Then imagine you burn 100 calories more each day by parking a bit further away from the entrance, climbing one flight of stairs, pacing on the phone, curling hand weights during TV watching. Painless, right? Over the course of the year, you would have achieved a calorie deficit of—are you ready?—91,250 calories. That means you just managed to lose 26 pounds in a single year, just with a few simple changes.

Now imagine you did that three years in a row. Need to lose 78 pounds? You just learned how.

Now imagine you decided to work even harder at it, focusing for even just 12 or 24 weeks on a medically supervised weight-loss program and remained focused on the small changes. You might lose 20, 30 or 40 pounds with a medically supervised plan or even more. So your weight loss in one year could be 50 pounds, and in three years could be 150 pounds.

You picked up this book because you want a solution to help you lose weight, which is probably the most important thing you can do to improve your health, your quality of life and your lifespan. Reading this book is an excellent start.

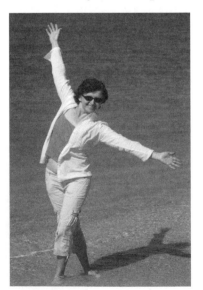

Remember that you *can* succeed. You *can* achieve your goals of losing weight and becoming the person you know you really are inside, becoming the new you.

It takes hard work. But you are worth it.

Don't wait. The time will never be just right.

—Napolean Hill

Losing weight doesn't mean you're never going to eat again. It doesn't even mean you're never going to eat anything that tastes good again. It just means you need to be careful of what you're eating. The following recipes are a sampling of those that can help you lose weight while still enjoying cooking a healthy, satisfying meal.

These recipes offered in this appendix are taken from Ditch Your Diet in 30 Days: 90 Easy, Healthy Meal and Snack Recipes for Effective Weight Loss by Chef Dave Fouts and Vicki Bovee, R.D. As the world's first Bariatric chef, Chef Dave received his culinary degree from Florida Culinary Institute in 1994 and is currently the corporate chef for the International Metabolic Institute (iMetabolic®) based in Reno, Nevada. Dr. Sasse founded International Metabolic Institute, a center offering sound medically supervised (nonsurgical) solutions for weight loss that involve dietary solutions, behavior-changing techniques, prescription weight-loss medications, fitness training, psychological counseling and inspirational life-coaching. See the Resources section of this book for more information on this center.

Cheddar, Bacon and Potato Breakfast Bake

Serves 4

4 ounces Canadian bacon, diced
½ small green bell pepper, diced
½ small red bell pepper, diced
1 small onion, chopped
1 cup egg substitute
½ pound russet potatoes, peeled and grated
½ cup sharp cheddar cheese, shredded
½ teaspoon black pepper
1 pinch salt, to taste

Directions

Preheat oven to 450. Spray a large quiche dish or 6 to 8 individual ramekins with nonstick cooking spray. Sauté Canadian bacon, peppers and onion until soft; drain on paper towels. Whisk egg substitute with potatoes, cheese, salt and pepper. Mix in Canadian bacon and vegetable mixture. Pour into prepared pan, spreading mixture evenly. Bake for 45 minutes, until center is set or until a knife inserted in the center comes out clean.

Nutrition Facts
Per serving
Calories 220   Calories from fat 70
Total fat 8g   Saturated fat 2g   Trans fat 0g
Cholesterol 15 mg
Sodium 660mg
Total carbohydrate 26g   Dietary fiber 3g
Sugars 11g   Protein 13g

Cheery Cherry Brunch Pie

Serves 6
½ pound turkey sausage
1 16-ounce can unsweetened tart cherries*, drained
½ cup low-fat cheddar cheese, shredded
1 cup reduced fat baking mix
1 teaspoon dried basil
1/8 teaspoon black pepper
4 large eggs
1-1/2 cups 1% milk

Directions

Preheat oven to 400. in a large skillet, cook sausage until brown, breaking into small pieces as it cooks; drain off fat. Remove from heat. Add cherries; mix well. Spoon sausage mixture into a 10-inch deep-dish pie plate; top with cheese. In a medium mixing bowl, combine baking mix, basil and pepper. Add eggs and milk; beat until smooth. Pour over cheese. Bake 35 to 40 minutes, or until a knife inserted in the center comes out clean.

Let cool for 5 minutes. Serve with a mixed green salad.

*Note: 1-1/2 cups frozen unsweetened tart cherries can be substituted for canned cherries. Partially thaw cherries, then coarsely chop and drain before adding to sausage.

Nutrition Facts
Per serving
Calories 250   Calories from fat 80
Total fat 8g   Saturated fat 2.5g
Cholesterol 155mg
Sodium 600mg
Total carbohydrate 25g   Dietary fiber 1g
Sugars 11g   Protein 18g

Mexican Scramble Breakfast Pita with Kiwi

Serves 2

2 large eggs
¼ teaspoon black pepper
2 small whole-wheat pitas, warmed
½ cup nonfat refried beans, warmed
¼ cup cooked diced potatoes, warmed
½ cup shredded iceberg lettuce
1 large sprig cilantro, chopped or sprig, for garnish
2 tablespoons salsa
2 each kiwi fruit, peeled and sliced

Directions

Scramble eggs with pepper. Cook over medium heat until thoroughly cooked. Fill warmed pita halves with warmed refried beans. Top with warmed potatoes and shredded lettuce. Add scrambled eggs, salsa and garnish with cilantro.

Serve 1 kiwi on the side per portion.

Nutrition Facts
Per serving
Calories 260   Calories from fat 45   Total fat 5g
Saturated fat 1.5 g
Cholesterol 180mg
Sodium 620mg
Total carbohydrate 41g   Dietary fiber 8g
Sugars 9g   Protein 14g

Banana Bran Muffins with Peanut Butter

Serves 24*

6 cups Grape-Nuts Flakes

5 cups whole-wheat flour

5 teaspoons baking soda

3 cups Splenda®

4 large eggs

1 quart low-fat buttermilk

1 teaspoon vanilla extract

1 cup unsweetened applesauce

6 large bananas, mashed

½ tablespoon natural peanut butter per muffin

Directions

Thoroughly mix all ingredients except the peanut butter. Bake fresh as needed. (Store in fridge for up to one week.) Fill muffin cups 2/3 full. Bake at 400 for 20 minutes.

One serving is two muffins and one tablespoon peanut butter.

*Note: Recipe yields 48 muffins or 24 servings.

Nutrition Facts

Per serving

Calories 300   Calories from fat 90   Total fat 10g

Saturated fat 1.5g

Cholesterol 35 mg

Sodium 430mg

Total carbohydrate 44g   Dietary fiber 6g

Sugars 10g   Protein 11g

Open-Face Turkey Avocado Sandwich with Grapes

Serves 1

1 slice whole-wheat bread
1-1/2 teaspoons light mayonnaise
½ medium avocado, peeled and sliced
2 ounces low sodium deli turkey
2 slices tomatoes
20 grapes

Directions
Spread mayo over bread and layer with turkey, tomatoes and avocado. Cut in half. Serve with grapes.

* * *

Nutrition Facts
Per serving
Calories 380 Calories from fat 170 Total fat 18g
Saturated fat 2g Cholesterol 30mg
Sodium 500mg
Total carbohydrate 43g Dietary fiber 10g
Sugars 19g Protein 19g

Shaved Ham, Turkey and Havarti Salad in Pita Pocket with Pineapple

Serves 4

4 ounces reduced sodium lean ham*, shaved
6 ounces low sodium turkey breast*, shaved
2 ounces havarti cheese, shredded
3 cups romaine lettuce, torn
2 small tomatoes, diced
½ medium cucumber, peeled and sliced
1 small green bell pepper, sliced
1 small onion, cut into rings
6 small radishes, thinly sliced
½ cup fresh parsley, chopped
1 clove garlic, crushed

Dressing

2 tablespoons olive oil
2 tablespoons lemon juice
1 teaspoon dried Italian seasoning
4 small-sized whole-wheat pita pockets
2 cups canned pineapple chunks in juice, drained

Directions

Combine ham, turkey, cheese, lettuce, tomatoes, cucumber, bell pepper, onion, radishes, parsley and garlic in large salad bowl. For dressing, whisk together in small bowl the olive oil, lemon juice and Italian seasoning. Stuff each small pita with salad mixture and drizzle with dressing. Serve each portion with ½ cup pineapple.

*Note: You may substitute shrimp, tuna or crab for this recipe.

Nutrition Facts
Per serving
Calories 350   Calories from fat 120   Total fat 14g
Saturated fat 5g   Cholesterol 45mg
Sodium 640mg
Total carbohydrate 38g   Dietary fiber 6g
Sugars 17g   Protein 22g

Mexican Chicken Wraps

Serves 6

2 medium tomatoes, chopped
1 4-ounce can green chilies, diced
1/3 cup green onions, sliced
1 tablespoon fresh cilantro, chopped
1 tablespoon canola oil
1 pound boneless skinless chicken breast, cut into 1-inch cubes
2 tablespoons water
1 ounce taco seasoning mix*
6 whole-wheat tortillas
6 tablespoons light sour cream

Directions

In a large bowl, combine tomatoes, chilies, green onions and cilantro; set aside. In a large skillet, heat oil over medium-high heat; add chicken and cook approximately 2 minutes. Add water and taco seasoning mix; continue to cook until chicken is cooked through. Mix in tomato mixture to skillet of seasoned chicken. Place ¼ cup filling on each tortilla; roll up. Garnish with 1 tablespoon sour cream.

*Note: Fillings may be prepared the night before, then wrapped in tortillas the next day.

. . . .

Nutrition Facts
Per serving
Calories 300   Calories from fat 70   Total fat 8g
Saturated fat 1g   Cholesterol 50mg
Sodium 590mg
Total carbohydrate 29g   Dietary fiber 3g
Sugars 3g   Protein 23g

Tex Mex Turkey Chili

Serves 8

2 pounds lean ground turkey

1 tablespoon olive oil

16 ounces canned tomatoes, chopped

2 cups onion, chopped

3 cloves garlic, chopped

¾ teaspoon salt

1 tablespoon chili powder

½ teaspoon dried oregano

½ teaspoon black pepper

1 bay leave

1 cup canned reduced sodium kidney beans

8 tablespoons light sour cream

8 tablespoons sharp cheddar cheese, shredded

Directions

In a large sauté pan, brown turkey in oil, stirring frequently. Add undrained tomatoes, onions, garlic, salt and remaining seasonings. Cover and simmer for 45 minutes. Stir in kidney beans. Cook for an additional 30 minutes; remove bay leaf.

To serve, divide into 8 equal portions and garnish each with 1 tablespoon cheese and 1 tablespoon light sour cream.

* * *

Nutrition Facts

Per serving

Calories 300 Calories from fat 144 Total fat 16g

Saturated fat 5g Cholesterol 03mg

Sodium 615mg

Total carbohydrate 14g Dietary fiber 4g

Sugars 10g Protein 25g

Balsamic Glazed Pork Tenderloin and Red Pepper Grits

Serves 4

3 cups low sodium chicken broth

¾ cup quick cooking grits, uncooked

2 tablespoons butter

1 clove garlic, minced

7 ounces roasted red peppers, drained and diced

1 pound lean pork tenderloin, cut into 4 equal portions

1/8 teaspoon black pepper

¼ cup balsamic vinegar

2 tablespoons honey

Directions

Bring broth to a boil. Add grits, butter and garlic, stirring with a whisk. Reduce heat and simmer, uncovered, for 5 minutes. Remove from heat; stir in red pepper. Cover and set aside.

While grits sit, heat a large nonstick skillet coated with cooking spray over medium-high heat. Add pork to pan; cook 4 minutes on each side or until done. Remove from pan.

Stir in vinegar and honey, scraping pan to loosen browned bits. Bring to a boil; cook 1 minute or until thick, stirring constantly with a whisk. Return pork to pan; turn to coat.

To serve, divide grits into 4 equal portions and place on plates. Add 1 piece of pork and evenly divide sauce over grits.

Nutrition Facts

Per serving

Calories 380   Calories from fat 100   Total fat 11g

Saturated fat 5g   Cholesterol 90mg

Sodium 290mg

Total carbohydrate 39g   Dietary fiber 1g

Sugars 13g   Protein 31g

Just for the Halibut Vegetable Stir-Fry With Baked Potato.

Serves 4

1 pound halibut steak, cut into 4 ounce steaks
1 medium tomato, diced
½ cup fresh mushrooms, sliced
½ cup onions, sliced
½ cup celery, diced
1 tablespoon lemon juice
2 teaspoons canola oil
¼ teaspoon thyme, ground
1/8 teaspoon salt
1 pinch black pepper
4 medium baked potatoes
8 teaspoons light tub margarine
4 teaspoons light sour cream

Directions

Preheat oven to 375. To cook potatoes, rinse and wrap with foil and place in oven for 45 minutes or until fork tender.

Sprinkle halibut with salt and pepper; place in a shallow baking dish. In large, preheated nonstick sauté pan add tomato, mushrooms, onion, celery, lemon juice, oil, thyme, salt and pepper; sauté until tender.

Spoon the vegetable mixture over halibut. Place covered halibut into oven and bake for 10 minutes or until halibut flakes when tested with a fork.

Serve each potato with 2 teaspoons margarine, 1 teaspoon light sour cream and halibut stir-fry.

Nutrition Facts
Per serving
Calories 390   Calories from fat 120   Total fat 13g
Saturated fat 2g   Cholesterol 40mg
Sodium 270mg
Total carbohydrate 39g   Dietary fiber 3g
Sugars 6g   Protein 28g

Spaghetti and Spinach Tomato Feta Pesto Bake

Serves 8

1 pound protein plus spaghetti, uncooked
10 ounces frozen chopped spinach, thawed and drained
½ cup parmesan cheese, grated
2 tablespoons water
8 ounces reduced fat feta cheese, crumbled
2 tablespoons reduced fat refrigerated pesto sauce
6 large plum tomatoes, cut into 2-inch pieces

Directions

Preheat oven to 350. Prepare pasta according to directions on package; drain. Toss cooked warm pasta with thawed spinach, parmesan cheese, water, feta cheese, plum tomatoes and pesto sauce.

Spray an 8x8 inch baking dish with nonstick cooking spray. Put pasta mixture into pan, cover with aluminum foil and bake for 20 minutes.

* * *

Nutrition Facts
Per serving
Calories 320   Calories from fat 70   Total fat 8g
Saturated fat 3g   Cholesterol 15mg
Sodium 530mg
Total carbohydrate 44g   Dietary fiber 6g
Sugars 4g   Protein 20g

Rum Marinated Beef Tenderloin and Cilantro Roasted Potatoes

Serves 6

Rum-marinated beef tenderloin

½ cup rum	2 cloves garlic, chopped
1 tablespoon olive oil	1 teaspoon ground oregano
1 tablespoon chili powder	¼ teaspoon hot pepper sauce

1-1/2 pounds beef tenderloin, cut into 6 4-ounce pieces

Tenderloin directions

Mix rum with next 5 ingredients for marinade. Marinate steaks in refrigerator for 30 minutes to 2 hours. Discard marinade once used. Grill streaks until medium rare.

Cilantro roasted potatoes

½ tablespoon olive oil	¾ pound potatoes, unpeeled and cut into wedges
½ tablespoon chili powder	½ medium onion, cut into thick wedges
1 teaspoon garlic, chopped	1-1/2 cups cherry tomatoes, halved
½ teaspoon salt	2 tablespoons cilantro, chopped
¼ teaspoon black pepper	2 tablespoons lime juice

Cilantro roasted potatoes directions

Preheat oven to 425. On a lightly oiled nonstick baking sheet, combine all seasoning ingredients. Add potatoes and onion; toss to coat evenly. Bake for 25 minutes.

Add tomatoes; bake an additional 7 to 10 minutes or until potatoes are tender. Transfer vegetables to large bowl; add cilantro. Sprinkle with lime juice; toss lightly.

* * *

Nutrition Facts

Per serving

Calories 390   Calories from fat 190   Total fat 22g

Saturated fat 8g   Cholesterol 100mg

Sodium 270mg

Total carbohydrate 13g   Dietary fiber 2g

Sugars 2g   Protein 32g

Chicken Carbinade With Couscous and Broccoli

Serves 8

1-1/2 pounds boneless skinless chicken breast, cut into 1-inch cubes

1-1/4 teaspoons salt	1 cup low sodium chicken broth
1 teaspoon black pepper	12 ounces nonalcoholic beer
4 tablespoons canola oil	2 bay leaves
4 large onions, sliced	1 teaspoon thyme
1 tablespoon tomato paste	1 tablespoon cider vinegar
2 cloves garlic, chopped	2 cups couscous, cooked
3 tablespoons all-purpose flour	4 cups broccoli florets, steamed

Directions

Preheat oven to 350. Pat chicken cubes dry; salt and pepper. In large sauté pan over medium-high heat add 2 tablespoons canola oil. When oil is heated sauté chicken in 3 batches; don't touch for 2 minutes to get a good sear. Set aside.

Add remaining oil over medium-low heat. Add onion and tomato paste; keep on medium-low for 5 minutes and stir. Turn heat up to medium and cook until golden brown. Add garlic to onions. Add flour; cook for 3 minutes. Add beef broth, chicken broth, beer, bay leaf, thyme and vinegar. Bring to a full simmer. Add chicken; place in oven for 2 to 2.5 hours with lid cracked.

To serve, divide into 8 equal portions and serve each with ¼ cup couscous and ½ cup steamed broccoli.

··

Nutrition Facts

Per serving

Calories 270   Calories from fat 80   Total fat 9g

Saturated fat 1g   Cholesterol 50mg

Sodium 480mg

Total carbohydrate 22g   Dietary fiber 3g

Sugars 4g   Protein 24g

Homemade Chicken Pot Pie Lasagna

Serves 10

12 pieces whole-wheat lasagna, uncooked
1 pound boneless skinless chicken breast, diced
3 cups fresh mushrooms, sliced
1 cup carrots, thinly sliced
½ cup green onions, sliced
1 cup frozen green peas, thawed and well drained

Directions

Prepare pasta according to package directions. Spray a large sauté pan with cooking spray; place over medium-high heat until hot. Add chicken and sauté 4 minutes or until cooked through. Drain well and set aside. Recoat sauté pan with cooking spray and place over medium-high heat until hot. Add mushrooms, carrots, green onions and peas; sauté 6 minutes. Set aside.

Sauce

½ cup all-purpose flour
3-1/2 cups nonfat milk
½ cup dry sherry
1 teaspoon dried thyme
½ teaspoon salt
¼ teaspoon cayenne pepper
15 ounces part-skim ricotta cheese
1-1/2 cups part-skim mozzarella cheese, grated and divided
½ cup reduced fat Swiss cheese, shredded

Sauce Directions

Preheat oven to 350. Place flour in a medium saucepan. Gradually add milk, stirring with a wire whisk until blended; stir in sherry. Bring to a boil over medium heat; cook for 5 minutes or until thickened, stirring constantly. Stir in thyme, salt and cayenne pepper. Reserve one cup of sauce and set aside.

In a bowl, combine ricotta cheese, 1 cup mozzarella and Swiss cheese. Spread 1 cup of the sauce over the bottom of a 13x9x2-inch pan.

Arrange 4 pieces of the lasagna (3 lengthwise, 1 widthwise) over the sauce. Top with half of ricotta cheese mixture, half of chicken mixture and half of remaining sauce mixture. Repeat layers, ending with 4 pieces of lasagna.

Spread reserved 1 cup of sauce over the last complete layer of lasagna, being sure to cover the lasagna completely. Cover lasagna with foil and bake for 1 hour. Uncover lasagna, sprinkle remaining ½ cup mozzarella cheese on top; bake an additional 5 minutes uncovered.

Re-cover and let stand 15 minutes before serving.

Nutrition Facts
Per serving
Calories 360   Calories from fat 80   Total fat 9g
Saturated fat 4.5 g   Cholesterol 50mg
Sodium 350mg
Total carbohydrate 37g   Dietary fiber 6g
Sugars 7g   Protein 31g

As always, you want to check with your own doctor before starting any kind of liquid diet replacement plan. This is especially true if you have special diet or health considerations, such as a history of eating disorders or diabetes. But in general, the program is safe for most people who are in reasonably good health and looking to jump-start their weight loss.

The iMetabolic® Meal Replacement Powder and protein bars can be ordered from www.iMetabolic.com.

Induction Meal Plan

An induction meal plan means nothing more than the kick-off to weight loss—no one expects you're going to spend the rest of your life eating nothing but 1,000 calories a day. But such a restricted caloric intake can have stunning weight-loss results—up to 40 pounds in 90 days (for more details, see my Web site offer at www.iMetabolic.com, where you can find a Weight Loss Success Starter Kit and a Special Report available for download).

Meal Plan 1 (Soy) 1,000 Calories

Time	Meal	Calories
Breakfast	2 scoops Bariatrix Essentials Meal Replacement Powder with 8 ounces nonfat milk	234
Mid-morning snack (choose one)	1 medium apple, pear, nectarine or peach OR 1 small orange, ½ banana OR 1 cup raspberries, blueberries or sliced strawberries	20-50
Lunch	2 scoops Bariatrix Essentials Meal Replacement Powder	234
	with 8 ounces nonfat milk, approved vegetables with 1 teaspoon oil/butter	140
Mid-afternoon snack	iMetabolic® Protein Bar OR Anytime Ready-to-Drink Shake Bar = 150-160 calories Shake = 100 calories (choose either bar or shake)	100-150
Dinner	iMetabolic® Meals To Go OR Meal Replacement Shake	234-300
	OR Lean Cuisine, Smart One or Healthy Choice Meal	(300 calories or less)

◇ Remember to track your TOTAL intake. You need to do the math, so you know exactly what each choice you make represents in caloric value. Mix and match your options so you stay at or under the 1,000-calorie limit.

◇ Include 1 serving of approved raw or cooked vegetables at lunch-time OR afternoon snack time above, the vegetables not to exceed 100 calories total for the day. You may add 1 teaspoon olive oil, canola oil or butter to your veggies (40 calories)—Total additional calories 140.

◇ If iMetabolic® Meal To Go meal or prepared meal is more than 300 calories, take off one of your snacks from your total daily intake—remember to do the math and stay under 1,000 calories.

◇ Take 1 multivitamin every day.

◇ Continue to drink a minimum of 8 glasses of water daily.

Weight (lbs)	\multicolumn{10}{c}{Height (ft)}
	4'9"	4'11"	5'1"	5'3"	5'5"	5'7"	5'9"	5'11"	6'1"	6'3"
154	33	31	29	27	26	24	23	22	20	19
165	36	33	31	29	28	26	24	23	22	21
176	38	36	33	31	29	28	26	25	23	22
187	40	38	35	33	31	29	28	26	25	24
198	43	40	37	35	33	31	29	28	26	25
209	45	42	40	37	35	33	31	29	28	26
220	48	44	42	39	37	35	33	31	29	28
231	50	47	44	41	39	36	34	32	31	29
243	52	49	46	43	40	38	36	34	32	30
254	55	51	48	45	42	40	38	35	34	32
265	57	53	50	47	44	42	39	37	35	33
276	59	56	52	49	46	43	41	39	37	35
287	62	58	54	51	48	45	42	40	38	36
298	64	60	56	53	50	47	44	42	39	37
309	67	62	58	55	51	48	46	43	41	39
320	69	64	60	57	53	50	47	45	42	40
331	71	67	62	59	55	52	49	46	44	42
342	74	69	65	61	57	54	51	48	45	43
353	76	71	67	63	59	55	52	49	47	44
364	78	73	69	64	61	57	54	51	48	46
375	81	76	71	66	62	59	56	52	50	47
386	83	78	73	68	64	61	57	54	51	48
397	86	80	75	70	66	62	59	56	53	50
408	88	82	77	72	68	64	60	57	54	51
419	90	84	79	74	70	66	62	59	56	53
430	93	87	81	76	72	67	64	60	57	54
441	95	89	83	78	73	69	65	62	59	55
452	98	91	85	80	75	71	67	63	60	57
463	100	93	87	82	77	73	69	65	61	58

Weight Category	BMI
Normal Weight	19 - 24.9
Overweight	25 - 29.9
Obese	30 - 38.9
Extreme Obesity	40 - 58

Resistance Training Program Instructions:

Cardiovascular Training

Cardiovascular training is critical to your ability to burn calories and improve cardiovascular capacity. There is such a wide range of potential processes to improve this capacity you will need to talk with your trainer to arrive at the most functional process for you to accomplish this important ingredient of your new lifestyle.

Exercise	Equipment, Location, Position
1. Chest press	Back of chair
2. Shoulder press	Under chair
3. Seated row	Around both doorknobs
4. Side raise	Under seat or standing
5. Leg squat	Squeeze glute muscles
6. Lunge	Doorway
7. Hamstring press	Doorknob
8. Leg extension	Chair leg
9. Triceps press down	Over top of door
10. Triceps press	Arms overhead
11. Arm curl	Elbows against sides
12. Abdominal crunch	Edge of chair

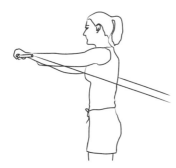

1. Chest Press: This exercise can be done either standing or seated, by winding the band around the back of a large chair. Bend elbows so hands are level with chest. With elbows at level height, press arms straight out in front of you, then slowly return to starting position.

Remember to use *slow* controlled movements.

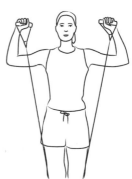

2. Shoulder Press: This exercise can be done standing or seated, by running band beneath chair seat (while seated) With arms at sides and bent 90 degrees at the elbow, slowly pull directly up, then slowly return to starting position.

3. Seated Row: This exercise can be done standing or seated in a chair. Wrap band around *both* doorknobs. Put arms out straight in front of you, slowly pull straight back, bending elbows and keeping them in close to your body. Slowly return to extended position.

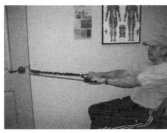
Position #1

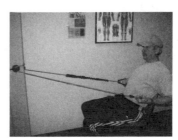
Position #2

4. Side Raise:
(this can also be done by standing on the band or by running it under the chair seat while seated.) Extend arm out straight at your side and at a 45-degree angle from front or back. Pull straight up to shoulder height and slowly return to starting position.

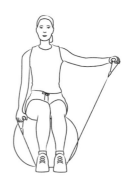

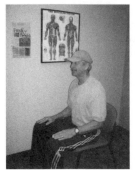

5. Leg Squat (the 25¢ squeeze): *This exercise does not use a band.* Begin in a standing position. Imagine you are squeezing a 25¢ piece between your glutes. Continue to pinch/clench those muscles as you slowly sit down (you don't want to drop that quarter!). As you sit, keep your head up and use the strength of your thighs to slowly lower yourself into your chair. Be sure your hands are in front of your shoulders. Make sure that your knees are over your feet and not extended over your toes during the squat. Rise back to your starting position.

6. Doorway Lunge:
Standing about 6 inches away from the entrance of a doorway, place your hands against the door frame with fingers pointing up and palm facing forward. Fingers should be at shoulder height. Stand close to the frame but leave enough room to step through the doorway entrance.

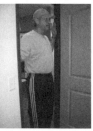 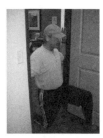

Position #1   Position #2

Lunge through the doorway with your left leg (coming down to a kneeling position with your right knee on the ground) while keeping your upper body upright and facing forward. Maintain your hand positions and place a small amount of pressure against the frame. Repeat with the right leg.

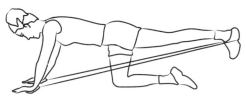

7. Hamstring Press—Version #1:
Get on your hands and knees and wrap a resistance band around the right foot. Hold the handles in each hand and begin the move with the right knee bent and flex the foot while extending the right leg straight back, squeezing the glutes. Return to starting position. Repeat on the opposite side.

Version #2, seated:
Make a lasso out of the band and loop it around your ankle. Loop the band around the doorknob on the same side of the door as the leg you are using. Hold band in hands and pull back to create tension. Start with leg in raised, straight position. Pull foot back down toward the floor. Repeat the process on the opposite leg.

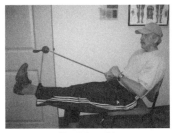 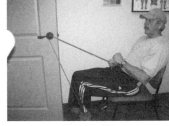

Position #1   Position #2

8. Leg Extension: Sit in chair. Make lasso out of band and loop around your ankle. Loop band around the front chair leg on the same side. Hold other end of band in hand on that side. Raise leg slowly until it is in a horizontal position. Slowly return foot to the floor. Repeat with the other leg.

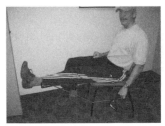 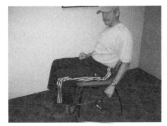

Position #1   Position #2

9. Triceps Kickback: Loop band over top of door frame. Grip handles firmly in each hand. Stand CLOSE to the edge of the door (if you're too far back, the band can slip off the top of the door and hit you in the face). Begin with elbows bent and band in a relaxed position. Slowly pull band down equally with both hands until arms are fully extended with hands toward the floor. Slowly return to starting position.

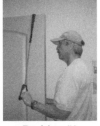 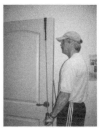

Position #1   Position #2

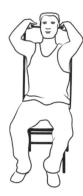

10. **Triceps Press:** Sit on band. With elbows bent, swing band so it comes up behind you. Slowly press band up until arms are straight, keeping elbows facing forward as you move up and back. Return to starting position.

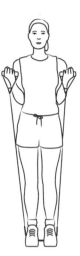

11. **Arm Curl:** Start by standing on the resistance band with one foot (less resistance) or with both feet (more resistance). Hold the handles to either side of your legs. Keeping your elbows tight to your sides, curl the resistance band to your shoulders without twisting your wrists. Return to starting position.

12. **Crunch:** Depending on your current strength, curls can be done from a seated position, where you simply slowly raise your knees toward your chest, to more active forms in which you are lying on the floor on your back and bringing your knees up to your chest. If you work with a trainer, then he or she can assign a movement equal to your current fitness level.

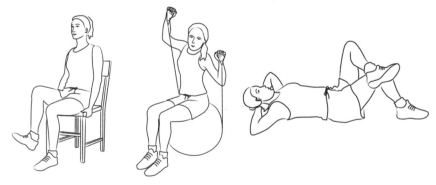

Appendix E—Rebound Weight Gain Blamed For Diets Failing

Sasse, K. (2008). *Rebound Weight Gain Blamed For Diets Failing*. Retrieved on Sept 16, 2008: http://www.emaxhealth.com/1/20037.html

Rebound Weight Gain Blamed For Diets Failing

Successful weight loss does not happen by magic, according to weight loss expert Dr. Kent Sasse. Rebound Weight Gain commonly occurs after a diet, and the pounds are put back on faster than they ever came off. And yet, some weight loss programs succeed while others fail.

"Diets don't work because they almost always lead to Rebound Weight Gain," says Dr. Sasse, founder and medical director of the International Metabolic Institute. "The loss of muscle and protein stores during dieting causes powerful biochemical signals that lead to intense hunger and weight gain after the diet comes to an end."

More than 50% of adults are significantly overweight, and many are dieting to lose those extra pounds. Medical weight loss centers like iMetabolic believe Rebound Weight Gain can be avoided with the right weight loss program. They note that diets alone don't work because they don't involve creating the right kind of calorie intake that can result in weight loss, appetite suppression, and maintenance of the muscle or protein mass. Nearly all diets result in depletion of muscle mass to an equal or greater degree than burning of the fat mass. When the diet comes to an end, the Rebound Weight Gain occurs as a result of the hunger and nutrient deprivation experienced by the muscles. Diets fail over time because they feel like deprivation to the dieter, and they require an unrealistic level of motivation to keep cutting calories. This does not last.

To avoid Rebound Weight Gain, medical experts recommend:

⬥ Cut calories while maintaining protein intake
⬥ Exercise five times a week during the diet and beyond to maintain muscle mass
⬥ Take multivitamins and drink plenty of water
⬥ Plan your transition back to real foods
⬥ Work with professionals on long-term behavior changes and appetite control
⬥ Consider a medically-supervised weight loss program, not just a diet

Most of us know that diets alone usually don't work for long because they are not sustainable as eating behaviors beyond a very short term. The right physician-supervised program can cut calories, utilize meal replacements, provide counseling and behavior tools, make use of appetite suppressing medications, and plan the transition to future phases of the program and a maintenance program. "It takes a comprehensive approach to avoid Rebound Weight Gain and succeed in long term weight loss," says Dr. Sasse.

Abers, S. *Mindful Eating 101*. (2006). Routledge

Albers, S. *Eating Mindfully*. (2003). New Harbinger Publications.

Andreyeva, T., Puhl, R.M. and Brownell, K.D. (2008). Changes in perceived weight discrimination among Americans, 1995-1996 through 2004-2006. *Obesity*.

Baechle, T.R., Earle, R.W. (2000). Essentials of strength training and conditioning-2nd Edition. *Human Kinetics*.

Blue, L. Obesity is contagious. *Time*: In partnership with CNN. Jul 25, 2007. Retrieved Sept 16, 2008 from http://www.time.com/time/health/article/0,8599,1646997,00.html?iid=sphere-inline-sidebar

Camie, B. Alcohol addiction and obesity. Published on 8/26/05 on buzzle.com: Intelligent life on the Web. Retrieved on 9/16/08 on, http://www.buzzle.com/editorials/8-26-2005-75508.asp

Elliot, S.S., Keim, N.L., Stern, J.S., Teff, K., Havel, P.J. (2002) Fructose, weight gain and the insulin resistance syndrome. *American Society for Clinical Nutrition*, 76, 911-922.

Fabricatore A.N., Wadden, T.A. (2003). Treatment of obesity: An overview. *Clinical Diabetes*, 21, 67-72.

Greenberg, J.A., Axen, K.V., Schnoll, R., Boozer, C.N. (2005). Coffee, tea and diabetes: the role of weight loss and caffeine. *Int J Obes* (Lond). 2005 Sep;29(9):1121-9.

Holt, S.H., Delargy, H.J., Lawton, C.L., Blundell, (1999). The effects of high-carbohydrates vs high-fat breakfast on feelings of fullness and alertness, and subsequent food intake. *International Journal of Food Science & Nutrition*, 50, 13-28.

Hu, F. B., Stampfer, M. J., Manson, J. E., Rimm, E., Colditz, G. A., Rosner, B. A., et al. (1997). Dietary fat intake and the risk of coronary heart disease in women. *N. Engl. J. Med*, 337(21), 1491-1499.

Hu, F.B., Willett, W.C. (2002). Optimal diets for prevention of coronary heart disease. *JAMA*, 288, 2569-2578.

Jacobson, M.F. (2005) Liquid Candy: How soft drinks are harming Americans' health. Center for Science in the Public Interest. Retrieved Jan 13, 2007, from http://www.cspinet.org/new/pdf/liquid_candy_final_w_new_supplement.pdf

Kissebah, A.H., Vydelingum, N., Murray, R., Evans, D.J., Hartz, A.J., Kalkhoff, R.K., et al. (1982). Relation of body fat distribution to metabolic complications of obesity. *Journal of Clinical Endocrinology & Metabolism*, 54, 254-260

Lambert, C. (2004). The way we eat now. *Harvard Magazine*. Retrieved Sept 16, 2008, from http://www.harvard-magazine.com/lib/04mj/pdf/0504-50.pdf

Levine, J.A.(2005). Measurement of energy expenditure. *Public Health Nutr.*, 8(7A), 1123-32. Review.

Levy, A.S., Heaton, A.W. (1993).Weight control practices of U.S. adults trying to lose weight. *Annals of Internal Medicine*, 19(7), 661-666. Retrieved Jan 13, 2008, from http://www.annals. org/cgi/content/full/119/7_Part_2/661

Ma, Y., Bertone, E.R., Stanek, E.J., Reed, J.W., Hebert, J.R., Cohen, N.L., et al. (2003). The association between eating patterns and obesity in a free living US population. *Am J Epidemiology,* 158, 85-92.

Malik, V.S., Schulze, M.B., Hu, F.B. (2006). Intake of sugar-sweetened beverages and weight gain: a systematic review. *Am J Clin Nutr*, 84, 274-288.

Mcgregor, W. (2007). Using portion size to cut calories. Weightlossforall.com, Retrieved Sept 16, 2008, from http://ezinearticles.com/?Using-Smart-Portion-Sizing-to-Cut-Calories&id= 539107&opt=print

Murase, T., Nagasawa, A., Suzuki, J., Hase, T., Tokimitsu, I. Beneficial effects of tea catechins on diet-induced obesity: stimulation of lipid catabolism in the liver. *Int J Obes Relat Metab Disord.* 2002 Nove;26(11):1459-64

Nielsen, S.J. (2003). Patterns and trends in food portion sizes (1977-1998). *JAMA*, 289(4),450-3.

Patel, S.R., Malhotra, A.,White, D.P., Gottieb, D.J., and Hu, F.B.(2006). Association between reduced sleep and weight gain in women. *Am J of Epidemiology*, 164(10), 947-954.

Puhl, R.M., Andreyeva, T., & Brownell, K.D. (2008). Perceptions of weight discrimination: prevalence and comparison to race and gender discrimination in America. *Int J Obes*, 1-9.

Sasse, K. (2008). Rebound weight gain blamed for diets failing. Emaxhealth.com/1/20037.html

Sasse, K. *Outpatient Weight-Loss Surgery: Safe and Effective Weight Loss with Modern Bariatric Surgery* (2009) 360 Publishing

Sasse, K. *After Weight Loss Surgery: Losing Weight, Avoiding Rebound Weight Gain, Overcoming Plateaus, and Maintaining a Healthy Weight for a Lifetime* (2009) 360 Publishing

Shamsuzzaman, A.S., Gersh, B.J., Somers, V.K. (2003). Obstructive sleep apnea: implications for cardiac and vascular disease. *Journal of the American Medical Association,* 290, 1906-1914

Spiegel, K., Tasall, E., Penev, P., Van Cauter, E. (2004). Sleep curtailment in healthy young men is associated with decreased Leptin levels, elevated Ghrelin levels, and increased hunger and appetite. *Annals of Internal Medicine,* 141(11), 846-857.

Standl, E., Bartnik, M., den Berghe, G.V., Betteridge, J., de Boer, M., Cosentino, F., et al. (2007). Guidelines on diabetes, pre-diabetes and cardiovascular diseases: full text: The Task Force on Diabetes and Cardiovascular Diseases of the European Society of Cardiology (ESC) and of the European Association for the Study of Diabetes (EASD), *European Heart Journal Supplements,* 9(C), C3-C74.

Story, M., French, S. (2004). Food advertising and marketing directed at Children and adolescent in the U.S. International *Journal of Behavioral Nutrition and Physical Activity,* 1(3): 1-17.

Vangsness, S. (2005). Mastering the mindful meal. Brigham and Women's hospital: Teaching affiliate of Harvard medical school. Retrieved Sept 16, 2008, from http://www. brighamandwomens.org/healtheweightforwomen/special_topics/ intelihealth0405.aspx?subID=submenu10#

Wansink, B. (2006). *Mindless Eating: Why We Eat More Than We Think*. New York: Bantam-Dell

Warner, J. (2005). Six secrets of successful weight loss. WedMD Health. Retrieved Sept 16, 2008, from http://www.medscape.com/ viewarticle/514752

Weigle, D.S., Duell, P.B., Connor, W.E., Steiner, R.A., Soules, M.R., Kuijper, J.L. (1997). Effect of fasting, refeeding and dietary fat restriction on plasma leptin levels. *J Clin Endocrinol Metab*, 82(2), 561-5.

Wolfram, S. Effects of green tea and EGCG on cardiovascular and metabolic health. *J Am Coll Nutr*, 2007 Aug;26(4):373S-388S. Review.

Yoshioka, M., St-Pierre, S., Drapeau, V., Dionne, I., Doucet, E., Suzuki, M., et al. (1999). Effects of red peppers on appetite and energy intake. *Br J Nutr*, 82(2), 115-123.

Food and Agriculture Organization, United Nations. Do Americans eat 3,790 calories per day? Diet blog: eat right get healthy. http://www.fao.org/statistics/yearbook/vol_1_2/pdf/United-States-of-America.pdf

Resources

Please note that this is only a partial list of resources that are considered the most relevant and salient to this particular publication. A more robust list of health and weight loss related resource information is available at www.sasseguides.com.

Websites: Obesity and Health

Aetna
www.intelihealth.com   *Sites mission is to empower people with trusted solutions for healthier lives. This is accomplished by providing credible information from the most trusted sources.*

eMedicineHealth
www.emedicinehealth.com   *Practical medical information is available wide ranging topics. With more than 5500 pages of health content, the site contains articles written by physicians for patients and consumers. eMedicineHealth also offers a RSS Feeds to alert viewers on new and updated content on the site.*

HealthCentral.com
www.healthcentral.com *Another in a series of robust sites offering content from Harvard Health Publications, A.D.A.M., HealthDay, and Thompson's PDR. The site also has a newsletter and a robust portal of other sites dedicated to obesity, nutrition, and other weight related issues.*

iMetabolic

www.iMetabolic.com *Practical weight-loss solutions including valuable information, programs and weight-loss protein snacks, shakes, and meal replacements. Contains informative sections on Diabetes and helpful weight loss calculators.*

MayoClinic.com

www.mayoclinic.com *More than 3,300 physicians, scientists, and researchers from Mayo Clinic share their expertise to empower you to manage your health. Site is complete with free newsletters and RSS feeds to alert viewers of specific content interests.*

Medscape

www.medscape.com *Site offers specialists, primary care physicians, and other health professionals the webs most robust and integrated medical information and educational tools. Site has the facility to deliver, automatically the reader specialty information that best fits his or her profile.*

Medline Plus

http://medlineplus.gov *Site brings together authoritative information from the National Library of Medicine (NLM), the National Institutes of Health (NIH), and other government agencies and health-related organizations. Preformulated searches are included in site and give easy access to medical journal articles. Site also has extensive information about drugs, an illustrated medical encyclopedia, interactive patient tutorials, and latest health news.*

Mayo Clinic
Education and Research

www.mayo.edu *Site explores the world of medical research and education at Mayo Clinic, to laboratory and clinical trials. Includes blogs and publications on a wide range of weight related topics.*

MedHelp

www.medhelp.org *Site contains over 15 years of accumulated information from doctors and other patients across hundreds of conditions. In addition, site has long-standing partnerships with the top medical institutions such as the Cleveland Clinic, National Jewish, Partners Health, and Mount Sinai.*

ObesityHelp

www.obesityhelp.com *Site was founded a peer support community to help those faced with life threatening morbid obesity. As of January 2008, over 600,000 people have become members on the ObesityHelp web site seeking help to find a solution to their weight loss problems.*

WebMD

www.webmd.com *The site blends expertise in medicine, journalism, health communication, and content creation to bring some of the most robust information possible. MedicineNet.com is a frequent contributor to WebMD and comprises the Medical Editorial Board. Site also has an independent medical review board that continuously oversees and reviews the site for accuracy and timeliness.*

Websites for the Latest in "Obesity" Related News

Naturalnews.com

www.naturalnews.com *Site is a non-profit collection of public education website covering topics that empower individuals to make positive changes in their health, environmental sensitivity, consumer choices, and informed skepticism.*

Medical News Today

www.medicalnewstoday.com *Site is updated with more than 150 articles on weekdays and over 40 articles at weekends. The website is divided into 117 medical categories/specialties, allowing one to browse only specific, relevant news. Advanced news archive searches allow access to over 100,000 archived articles.*

National Institutes of Health

www.health.nih.gov *The National Institutes of Health (NIH) is part of the U.S. Department of Health and Human Services, and acts as the primary Federal agency for conducting and supporting medical research. NIH scientists investigate ways to prevent disease as well as the causes, treatments, and even cures for common and rare diseases. Composed of 27 Institutes and Centers, the NIH provides leadership and financial support to researchers in every state and throughout the world.*

Centers for Disease Control and Prevention

www.cdc.gov *CDC.gov provides users with credible, reliable health information on; data and statistics, diseases and conditions, emergencies and disasters, environmental health, healthy living, life stages, and a plethora of other information related to health and wellness.*

MedicineNet.com

www.medicinenet.com *Site is an online, healthcare media publishing company. It provides easy-to-read, in-depth, authoritative medical information for consumers. Medical information is doctor-generated by a network of over 70 U.S. Board Certified physicians.*

Government Organizations

Food and Nutrition Service

United States Department of Agriculture
Food & Nutrition Service
3101 Park Center Dr., Alexandria, VA 22302
www.fns.usda.gov/fns
The Food and Nutrition Service (FNS), formerly known as the Food and Consumer Service, administers the nutrition assistance programs of the U.S. Department of Agriculture. One of their primary goals is to "Improve the Nation's Nutrition and Health"

National Institutes of Health

9000 Rockville Pike, Bethesda, MD 20892
301-496-4000
www.nih.gov
The National Institutes of Health (NIH) is part of the U.S. Department of Health and Human Services, and acts as the primary Federal agency for conducting and supporting medical research. NIH scientists investigate ways to prevent disease as well as the causes, treatments, and even cures for common and rare diseases. Composed of 27 Institutes and Centers, the NIH provides leadership and financial support to researchers in every state and throughout the world.

Office of the Surgeon General (OSG)
Department of Health & Human Services
Office of the Surgeon General
5600 Fishers Ln., Rm. 18-66, Rockville, MD 20857
301-443-4000
www.surgeongeneral.gov
The Surgeon General serves as America's chief health educator by providing Americans the best scientific information available on how to improve their health and reduce the risk of illness and injury. The Surgeon General is appointed by the President of the United States with the advice and consent of the United States Senate for a 4-year term of office.

Weight-Control Information Network (WIN)
One WIN Wy., Bethesda, MD 20892-3665
877-946-4627
www.win.niddk.nih.gov
WIN was established in 1994 to provide the general-public, health professionals, the media, and Congress with up-to-date, science-based information on obesity, weight control, physical activity, and related nutritional issues.

Foundation for the National Institutes of Health
9650 Rockville Pike, Bethesda, MD 20814-3999
301-402-5311
www.fnih.org
The Foundation for the National Institutes of Health was established by the United States Congress to support the mission of the National Institutes of Health (NIH): improving health through scientific discovery.

The National Weight Control Registry
Brown Medical School/The Miriam Hospital
Weight Control & Diabetes Research Center
196 Richmond St., Providence, RI 02903
800-606-6927
www.nwcr.ws
Given the prevailing belief that few individuals succeed at long-term weight loss, the NWCR was founded to identify and investigate the characteristics of individuals who have succeeded at long-term weight loss. The NWCR is tracking over 5,000 individuals who have lost significant amounts of weight and kept it off for long periods.

Calorie Control Council
www.caloriecontrol.org
Provides information on cutting calories and fat in ones diet, tips on achieving and maintaining a healthy weight, understanding common low-calorie, reduced-fat foods and beverages (and the ingredients that make them possible.

The President's Council on Physical Fitness and Sports
Department of Health and Human Services
PCPFS, Department W, 200 Independence Ave., S.W., Rm. 738-H
Washington, D.C. 20201
202-690-9000
www.fitness.gov
Site represents the health, physical activity, fitness and sports information web site dedicated by the President's Council on physical fitness and sports.

Bariatric

American Society for Metabolic & Bariatric Surgery
100 SW 75th St., Ste. 201, Gainesville, FL 32607
352-331-4900
www.asbs.org
The purpose of the society is to advance the art and science of bariatric surgery by continued encouragement of its members to carry out the following mission: to improve the care and treatment of people with obesity and related diseases.; to advance the science and understanding of metabolic surgery; to foster communication between health professional on obesity and related conditions; to be the recognized authority and resource on metabolic and bariatric surgery; and to advocate for health care policy that ensures patient access to high quality prevention and treatment of obesity.

American Society of Bariatric Physicians (ASBP)
2821 South Parker Rd., Ste. 625, Aurora, CO 80014
303-770-2526
www.asbp.org
The American Society of Bariatric Physicians is a leading national professional organization providing physicians and other health professionals with education in the medical management of weight loss and related medical conditions. Bariatric Medicine is defined as the art and science of medical weight management and associated co-morbidities.

Diabetes

State of Diabetes Complications in America
888-825-5249
www.stateofdiabetes.com
This website is part of a national education program called the State of Diabetes Complications in America, created by the American Association of Clinical Endocrinologists (AACE) in partnership with

the members of the diabetes complications consortium, including the Amputee Coalition of America (ACA), Mended Hearts, National Federation of the Blind (NFB) and the National Kidney Foundation (NKF). The consortium was formed to provide beneficial information to people with type 2 diabetes about how to reduce the risk of the health complications associated with the disease, as well as support and encouragement to people who have experienced these serious health problems.

National Diabetes Education Program

One Diabetes Wy., Bethesda, MD 20814-9692

301-496-3583

www.ndep.nih.gov

The National Diabetes Education Program is a federally-funded program sponsored by the U.S. Department of Health and Human Services' National Institutes of Health and the Centers for Disease Control and Prevention and includes over 200 partners at the federal, state and local levels, working together to improve the treatment and outcomes for people with diabetes, promote early diagnosis, and prevent or delay the onset of type 2 diabetes.

Joslin Diabetes Center

One Joslin Place, Boston, MA 02215

617-732-2400

www.joslin.org

Joslin Diabetes Center is the only diabetes institution in the world that goes beyond a single focus. With efforts in these three critical areas, a synergy develops: researchers, clinicians and educators collaborate in ways that produce cutting-edge scientific discovery, unique clinical care models and pioneering educational strategies. This one-of-a-kind framework has an impact on people with diabetes locally, nationally and across the globe.

Juvenile Diabetes Research Foundation International

120 Wall St., New York, NY 10005-4001

800-533-2873

www.jdrf.org

JDRF is the leader in research leading to a cure for type 1 diabetes in the world. It sets the global agenda for diabetes research, and is the largest charitable foundation and advocate of diabetes science worldwide.

Nutrition

Society for Nutrition Education (SNE)

9100 Purdue Rd., Ste. 200, Indianapolis, IN 46268

317-328-4627

www.sne.org

SNE is dedicated to promoting effective nutrition education and communication to support and improve healthful behaviors and has a vision of healthy communities through nutrition education and advocacy.

Nutrition.Gov

National Agricultural Library

Food and Nutrition Information Center

Nutrition.gov Staff, 10301 Baltimore Ave., Beltsville, MD 20705-2351

www.nutrition.gov

Site is designed to allow users' access to practical information on healthy eating, dietary supplements, fitness and how to keep food safe. The site is updated with the latest news and features links to interesting sites.

American Society for Nutrition
9650 Rockville Pike, Bethesda, MD 20814
301-634-7050
www.nutrition.org
The American Society for Nutrition (ASN) is a non-profit organization dedicated to bringing together the world's top researchers, clinical nutritionists and industry to advance the knowledge and application of nutrition for the sake of humans and animals. Focus ranges from the most critical details of research and application to the broadest applications in society, in the United States and around the world.

Obesity

North American Association for the Study of Obesity (NAASO)
The Obesity Society (AOA), 8630 Fenton St., Ste. 814, Silver Spring, MD 20910
301-563-6526
www.obesity.org
The Obesity Society is the leading scientific society dedicated to the study of obesity. Since 1982, The Obesity Society has been committed to encouraging research on the causes and treatment of obesity and to keeping the medical community and public informed of new advances.

Women's Health

National Women's Health Resource Center
157 Broad St., Ste. 106, Red Bank, NJ 07701
800-986-9472
www.healthywomen.org
The site provides women in-depth, objective, physician-approved information on a broad range of women's health issues. With more than 100 topics in its health library, including the latest medical advancements in each field, the site offers a robust level of support for females.

Womenshealth.Gov
U.S. Department of Health & Human Services
800-994-9662
www.womenshealth.gov
The Office on Women's Health (OWH) was established within the U.S. Department of Health and Human Services. Its Vision is to ensure that "All Women and Girls are Healthier and Have a Better Sense of Well Being." Its mission is to "provide leadership to promote health equity for women and girls through sex/gender-specific approaches.

Sister to Sister: The Women's Heart Health Foundation
4701 Willard Ave., Ste.223, Chevy Chase, MD 20815
301-718-8033
www.sistertosister.org
Sister to Sister is a 501(c)(3) nonprofit foundation dedicated to preventing heart disease in women. The organization's goal is to promise women that they have the power to protect their own hearts.

Women's Health Initiative (WHI)
2 Rockledge Ctr., Ste. 10018, MS 7936 6701, Rockledge Dr., Bethesda, MD 20892-7936
301-402-2900
www.nhlbi.nih.gov/whi
The Women's Health Initiative (WHI) represents a major 15-year research program to address the most common causes of death, disability and poor quality of life in postmenopausal women – cardiovascular disease, cancer, and osteoporosis.

Women's Heart Foundation

P.O. Box 7827, West Trenton, NJ 08628

609-771-3778

www.womensheart.org

Women's Heart Foundation is the only non-governmental organization that implements heart disease prevention projects. It consists of a coalition of executive nurses, civic leaders, community health directors, hospitals, women's heart centers, partners, providers and corporate sponsors responding to the health crisis of women's heart disease and the urgent need for prevention programs. WHF advocates for women and supports early intervention and excellence of care of women.

MGH Center for Women's Mental Health

Perinatal and Reproductive Psychiatry Program Simches Research Building

185 Cambridge St., Ste. 2200, Boston, MA 02114

617-724-7792

www.womensmentalhealth.org

Site provides a range of current information including discussion of new research findings in women's mental health and how such investigations inform day-to-day clinical practice. Despite the growing number of studies being conducted in women's health, the clinical implications of such work are frequently controversial, leaving patients with questions regarding the most appropriate path to follow. Providing these resources to patients and their doctors so that individual clinical decisions can be made in a thoughtful and collaborative fashion.

DOCTOR'S ORDERS

About the Author

Kent Sasse, MD, MPH, FACS, is a nationally renowned authority on surgical weight-loss procedures and a leader in the rapidly evolving field of bariatric surgery. The distinguished recipient of several awards, including membership in the prestigious Alpha Omega Alpha Society for top medical graduates in the country, Dr. Sasse is founder and medical director of both the iMetabolic International Metabolic Institute and Western Bariatric Institute, a nationally recognized ASMBS Center of Excellence.

The recipient of a bachelor's degree in biochemistry at the University of California San Diego, where he graduated cum laude, and two master's degrees, including a master's degree in public health stemming from research related to biostatistics and bioethics, from the University of California Berkeley, Dr. Sasse completed residency training in surgery, focusing on gastrointestinal surgery and physiology, at the University of California San Francisco, as well as fellowship training at the Lahey Clinic in Boston, Massachusetts, before establishing his practice in northern Nevada.

Dedicated to the highest levels of scientific research and individualized, state-of-the-art treatment of patients, Dr. Sasse brings a wealth of experience and expertise to the rapidly evolving field of weight-loss surgery. He has written and continues to pursue several IRB-approved research protocols regarding weight loss and weight-loss surgery, and he lectures frequently on topics related to obesity and weight reduction at the University of Nevada School of Medicine. Through his nationally recognized programs, Dr. Sasse and his outstanding faculty provide patients the highest levels of compassionate medicine, scientific evidence, and personalized care in the field of weight reduction.

Dr. Sasse was, until recently, a United States Air Force 9026th Air Reserve Squadron attending surgeon at the Malcolm Grow Medical Center located at Andrews Air Force Base in Maryland. He is the author of numerous books and publications, audio programs, newsletters and a Web site, and is a featured national speaker in the field of weight-loss, bariatric medicine and weight-loss surgical procedures. He lectures frequently at the University of Nevada School of Medicine on topics related to weight loss and obesity.

Dr. Sasse is the founder of the Obesity Prevention Foundation, a nonprofit foundation dedicated to the prevention of obesity and excessive weight gain in children. Together with Drs. Robert Watson, John Ganser and Mark Kozar, the Foundation performs school programs and outreach to parents, teachers and kids to provide tools to prevent obesity. Visit www.ObesityPrevention.org to learn more.

Please visit www.sasseguide.com for more information on Dr. Sasse and his world-renowned programs and facilities.